D0953183

DIAGNOSED WITH FIBROIDS?
LEARN THE FACTS:

- Fibroids are not cancer, they don't cause cancer, and they do not even increase the risk of having cancer

- Fibroids have a tendency to run in families, and women who have never had children are more likely to develop them

- Watchful waiting is the BEST strategy, unless you already have symptoms that need treatment

- Other conditions can be mistaken for fibroids: adenomyosis, ovarian cysts, and uterine polyps

- Most women with fibroids can get pregnant and carry to term without difficulty

- Fibroids can stabilize or shrink, especially after menopause

- Drugs can sometimes shrink fibroids and control symptoms but may be harmful if used long term

- Stress levels can affect fibroids.

Up to 40 percent of women between the ages of 25 and 45 have uterine fibroids and each one faces this question: "What should I do?" Make the choice that's right for you.

Find out . . .

WHAT YOUR DOCTOR MAY *NOT* TELL YOU ABOUT FIBROIDS

WHAT YOUR DOCTOR MAY *NOT* TELL YOU ABOUT
FIBROIDS

New Techniques and Therapies–Including

Breakthrough Alternatives to Hysterectomy

SCOTT C. GOODWIN, M.D.
professor, Department of Radiological Sciences,
UCLA School of Medicine

MICHAEL BRODER, M.D.
assistant professor, Department of Obstetrics and Gynecology,
UCLA School of Medicine

and DAVID DRUM

FOREWORD BY CARLA DIONNE
executive director, National Uterine Fibroids Foundation

WARNER BOOKS

An AOL Time Warner Company

The information herein is not intended to replace the services of trained health professionals. You are advised to consult with your health care professional with regard to matters relating to your health, and in particular regarding matters that may require diagnosis or medical attention.

The title of the series What Your Doctor May *Not* Tell You About . . . and the related trade dress are trademarks owned by Warner Books, Inc., and may not be used without permission.

Warner Books, Inc., 1271 Avenue of the Americas, New York, NY 10020

Visit our Web site at www.twbookmark.com

 An AOL Time Warner Company

Printed in the United States of America

First Printing: April 2003
10 9 8 7 6 5 4 3 2 1

Library of Congress Cataloging-in-Publication Data
Goodwin, Scott C.
    What your doctor may not tell you about fibroids : new techniques and therapies—including breakthrough alternatives to hysterectomy / Scott C. Goodwin, Michael Broder, and David Drum.
        p. cm.
    Includes bibliographical references and index.
    ISBN 0-446-67853-8
    1.Uterine fibroids—Popular works, I. Broder, Michael S., M.D. II. Drum, David. III. Title.
RC280.U8 G58 2003
616.99'366—dc21   2002033116

Cover design by Diane Luger
Book design by Charles A. Sutherland

Acknowledgments

I am grateful to so many for their contributions to this book: First and foremost to my wife, Suzie, and my sons, Alexander and Adam, for their support and patience during my absences these past six years since the advent of uterine fibroid embolization; to my coauthors, Dr. Michael Broder and Mr. David Drum, for doing the heavy lifting on this book; to our agent, Nancy Crossman, for shepherding a three-way collaboration; to our editor at Warner Books, Diana Baroni, for her many helpful and substantive suggestions; to Wendy Landow, the managing director at the Cardiovascular and Interventional Radiology Research and Education Foundation for her relentless pursuit of excellence in the research of uterine fibroid embolization; to Dr. James Spies, the vice chairman of radiology at Georgetown for helping me to be a better scientist; and to Carla Dionne, technical writer extraordinaire, the executive director of the National Uterine Fibroids Foundation for her tireless work on behalf of women with fibroids and for her extensive work on this book, without which it would be a mere shadow of what it is now.

Scott C. Goodwin, M.D.

This book would not have been possible without the help and support of many people. My wife, Donna, and my children, Noah, Maya, and Jacob, provided a touchstone during many long months spent writing this book. I would also like to thank my coauthors, Scott Goodwin and David Drum, for their dedication to getting this right; my agent, Nancy Crossman, for her tireless help in this and other endeavors; Kim Mowrey, who at times put aside work on his own manuscript to help me finish this one; and Carla Dionne, without whose voice many women with uterine fibroids would be unheard.

Michael S. Broder, M.D.

Contents

Foreword

Only a few short years ago very little published information on uterine fibroids and treatment options was available to the general public. Furthermore, the few books that were offered typically focused on hysterectomy (instead of uterine fibroids) and often presented conflicting and confusing advice based more on personal theories, anecdotal evidence, and surgical and practice preferences of a single physician than on scientific medical research. From this, along with the advice of their physicians, women were faced with making potentially life-altering decisions about how to treat their fibroids.

Recently, a thorough review of the medical research on uterine fibroids was launched at the Duke University Evidence-Based Practice Center. The intention was to review all of the currently available evidence on the benefits, risks, and costs of commonly used medical and invasive therapies for uterine fibroids and to develop a list of recommendations for future research. As it turned out, this thorough review of the published medical literature painted a rather disappointing and dismal picture of uterine fibroids research. The detailed remarks in the Findings section of this report used the following language to describe what the investigators uncovered:

- The majority of the articles . . . do not provide sufficient information . . .
- Data were sparse . . .
- Data are lacking . . .
- Data are limited . . .
- There are no data . . . (this phrase appeared five times)
- Data are insufficient . . . (this phrase appeared three times)
- . . . exact relationship is unclear . . .
- . . . there is a remarkable lack of randomized trial data . . .
- . . . there is a lack of prospective data . . .
- . . . the current state of the literature does not permit definitive conclusions . . .
- . . . additional studies are needed . . .
- In general, there was a remarkable lack of high quality evidence supporting the effectiveness of most interventions for symptomatic fibroids.

As a woman, if you have been confused and uncertain about your treatment options for your fibroids, then this report clearly showed that you have good reason to be! Unmistakably, lack of research on uterine fibroids represents an incredible void in the field of women's health.

Given the lack of solid medical science on uterine fibroids and treatments, what is a woman diagnosed with these tumors supposed to do? Over a million women will be diagnosed with uterine fibroids in the United States this year, and each one of them will be facing this question and attempting to answer it without solid evidence to support any decision she may make about treatment.

Thankfully, the authors of this book, Scott Goodwin, M.D., and Michael Broder, M.D., have pulled together a comprehensive guide on uterine fibroids and treatments, old and new. Their discussion of each element of related information takes into account both the patient and physician perspectives and considers the risks and benefits of each possible road a woman may choose to walk down for treatment of her fibroids. They recognize the current lack of well-designed research and discuss the shortcomings, as well as the strong points, of the limited studies that have been done. Hopefully, the contents of this book will help you navigate the minefield of incomplete and inaccurate information that is often shared with a patient during discussions of treatment options for fibroids.

In 1998, after more than a decade of suffering from uterine fibroids, uterine fibroid embolization (UFE) gave me my quality of life back by putting an end to abnormal bleeding, urinary incontinence, pelvic pressure, back pain, and continued fibroid growth. However, my decision to undergo UFE was based on limited research information, as this fibroid treatment was still in early research stages in the United States at that time. How or why would I choose this procedure when so little published research information was available? As someone who had desperately tried to learn as much as possible about naturopathic remedies, medical therapies (prescribed drugs), hysterectomy, and myomectomy, I already knew precisely what Duke University was going to uncover with their Evidence-Based Practice Center study of uterine fibroids: "The majority of the articles . . . do not provide sufficient information . . .".

Yet, with highly symptomatic fibroids, I required treatment. It's a sad statement to make, but from my perspective and *based on the research,* UFE was no worse than any other treatment choice available. Today I'm happy to say that it was the best health care decision I could have made at the time. I do not regret my decision to undergo UFE and would choose this treatment option again, if need be. With time, research has shown it to be a highly effective treatment with tremendous success and limited risks to the patient. Even so, we still need to learn more—just as we need to learn more about alternative treatments, medical therapies, myomectomy, and hysterectomy. Perhaps in our pursuit of more research on uterine fibroids, we'll even uncover a better treatment than all of those currently available.

In the meanwhile over a million women this year will be diagnosed with fibroids and in search of accurate and appropriate information to help them understand their disease. Many of these women may need to make a treatment decision now. If you are one of the women with symptomatic fibroids who simply cannot wait for what the future of research holds on uterine fibroids, then this book will guide you through the maze of information you need to know in order to enhance your quality of life through lifestyle changes and make an informed decision about treatments currently available.

Carla Dionne
Executive Director
National Uterine Fibroids Foundation
Author, *Sex, Lies & the Truth About Uterine Fibroids*

Introduction

SCOTT C. GOODWIN, M.D.

How does an interventional radiologist end up writing a book about uterine fibroids? The story began on Thanksgiving Day in 1994. I was on call at UCLA and received a page from the Department of Obstetrics and Gynecology about a patient who was having severe bleeding after myomectomy. We brought her down to Radiology and embolized her uterine arteries. Embolization is a procedure that eliminates the blood flow to the uterine arteries. Her bleeding stopped immediately, and her vital signs stabilized. Although embolization had been used for decades to stop bleeding after childbirth or gynecologic surgery, this case affirmed its importance to me and the referring physician.

The next piece of the puzzle dropped into place in 1995 when Dr. Ravina and his colleagues in France published the first report of treating fibroids with uterine artery embolization. We started our program in 1996 and presented our early results at the 1997 Society of Cardiovascular and Interventional Radiology annual meeting. The response to that presentation astounded me. Women came from the world over to have embolization to save their uteri and/or avoid major surgery. Virtually every major media outlet carried the story including television and radio stations, newspapers, and magazines. I was asked nearly one hundred times to lecture on embolization at national and international meetings.

Eventually the idea of this book came into being. I knew that the book would be more complete if an obstetrician and gynecologist was a coauthor. Happily, Dr. Michael Broder agreed to write the book with me. Over the years, I have collaborated with several obstetricians and gynecologists. What has impressed me about Dr. Broder is his evidence-based approach to medicine. Simply put, he wants to do what is in the patient's best interest based on the available scientific evidence with no regard to personal gain.

Most, but not all, physicians take their fiduciary responsibility to their patients very seriously. Once, following a lecture on fibroid embolization to an obstetrician and gynecologist group, I asked one of the physicians why there was so much resistance to embolization in the obstetrician and gynecologist community. He told me that gynecologists consider fibroids an annuity. He related that in today's managed care environment physicians receive relatively little for deliveries and routine visits—the only significant payday is the hysterectomy.

The most important thing I have learned from my experiences with women with fibroids is that removing the uterus of approximately three hundred thousand women per year in the United States for benign disease is simply not acceptable. The most significant contribution the development of uterine fibroid embolization has made, in my opinion, is to serve as a wake-up call to researchers and clinicians to come up with something better than the scalpel. Hopefully, some day hysterectomy, myomectomy, and embolization will all be paragraphs on a page of a medical history textbook. When fibroids as a whole are understood well enough, noninvasive treatments will be developed. Ultimately, our goal as physicians ought to be to put ourselves out of business.

MICHAEL S. BRODER, M.D.

I didn't begin my career as a gynecologist specializing in uterine fibroids. I really had no intention of helping women find alternatives to hysterectomy for this common condition. I did my residency in obstetrics and gynecology at UCLA and then started a fellowship in an area of research that deals with measuring and improving the quality of health care. During the course of the fellowship, I became involved in a research project at the RAND Corporation. You may know of the RAND Corporation because of its involvement in military and government policy planning. The truth is, RAND does far more health-related research now than it does military research. RAND is a think tank, and one type of health care research that originated there is sometimes called "appropriateness" work. These types of studies involve picking a procedure or a condition and examining medical records or interviewing patients to determine whether those patients received the ideal care for that condition. In 1996 I joined a group of researchers who had started doing this type of study about hysterectomy. While past research had examined the appropriateness of hysterectomies, this one was a little different. We took a very in-depth look at almost five hundred women who had had hysterectomies at a variety of medical centers in Southern California. We reviewed each medical record and spoke to every patient.

What we learned was shocking even to us. We found that more than seven out of ten women did not have adequate evaluations before they were told they needed hysterectomy. Seven out of ten. We checked and rechecked our results but couldn't come to any other conclusion. The quality of care for women who have hysterectomies is entirely inadequate. We published our results in the *Journal of Obstetrics and Gynecology* in 2000. The response was overwhelming. Many, many gynecologists were sure we had done something wrong or that our methods were flawed. Many patients were sure we were right. My office began to overflow with women who had been told they needed hysterectomies and who wanted my opinion about whether this was the right step.

Sadly, I found that the results of my study played out in my practice as well. About one-third of the women I saw not only didn't need hysterectomies, but in my opinion they didn't need anything at all—not medications, not more tests, not anything. Their doctors had recommended hysterectomies for conditions that were not causing these women any problems and were not likely to any time in the near future. Another third of the women probably needed something, but hysterectomy certainly wasn't their only option. Finally, about one-third did seem to be best served by hysterectomy. But even these women benefited by a discussion of the other potential options and why their condition really could be best treated with hysterectomy.

Because fibroids are one of the most common reasons for hysterectomy, I started seeing more and more patients with uterine fibroids, and many of them tell the same story. The doctor diagnoses them with fibroids and tells them the only solution is a hysterectomy. Many women take this at face value and submit to the operation. A few others search and search for other options; some find what they need, some do not. The lucky ones learn through this process that how to treat fibroids is *their* choice, not their doctor's. This is a liberating realization, but not nearly enough women reach this level of understanding.

If you have uterine fibroids, hysterectomy is not the only option. Alternative treatments, both invasive and non-invasive, do exist. Uterine fibroids are a benign condition. For many women, just the knowledge that they do not have cancer and that their fibroids can be watched is treatment enough.

The body is an amazing piece of machinery, but it is more than a machine. In a car, we know that brakes have one function (an important function, but still only one function). The body is not that simple. It is true that the main function of the uterus is bearing children. However, it is presumptuous to assume that one function is everything. Some studies suggest that the uterus secretes its own hormones that interact with the ovaries and perhaps other organs in the body. Perhaps there are more functions of the uterus that remain unknown. But without good evidence that the uterus is useless beyond childbearing, we ought to try our best to leave it where it is.

Many women try to find a doctor who is willing to listen to their concerns and end up disappointed. Too many doctors take the position that only a doctor can decide whether a uterus stays in or comes out. The truth is that nobody is more invested in medical treatment than the patient herself.

I want women to know the history of the treatment of fibroids; to know about the various experimental and investigational techniques; and to understand the issues surrounding alternative medications, exercise, and other ways to treat fibroids. This book is aimed at giving women with a new diagnosis of uterine fibroids all the information they need to make informed decisions. Only when patients are truly partners with their doctors can the best outcome be ensured.

Primum no nocere. "First, do no harm."
—*Hippocrates*

WHAT YOUR DOCTOR
MAY *NOT* TELL YOU
ABOUT
FIBROIDS

Chapter 1

Fibroids

One summer day in Atlanta, Georgia, an attractive businesswoman named Victoria emerged from her doctor's office. The well-dressed forty-year-old seemed composed, but inside she was in turmoil. She had just seen her gynecologist because of some puzzling and excessive vaginal bleeding. She came out with an unexpected diagnosis of uterine fibroids.

Victoria stepped into the elevator and pushed the "down" button. She didn't know anything about fibroids. Her gynecologist told her she had "at least one" growing inside her uterus. It was the size of a tennis ball, perhaps. "For now, let's just watch it," her doctor said. Victoria trusted her doctor, who explained medical issues in a frank, matter-of-fact way. However, her doctor said that if the fibroids continued growing, Victoria would need a hysterectomy. The word was like a depth charge inside her. The idea that her uterus might be surgically removed from her body sent a primitive ripple of fear through her, and she involuntarily shuddered as she got off the elevator and walked outside into the bright afternoon sun.

It seemed to Victoria as though her entire body was suddenly under attack. She was afraid of fibroids. She feared cancer. She didn't want surgery. She didn't want

> to lose her uterus. She wanted children. The prospect
> of a hysterectomy seemed at that moment to roll to-
> ward her like a wild, unstoppable freight train.
>
> Unlocking the door to her car, Victoria burst into
> tears.

Fibroids are small, noncancerous growths that appear in the vast majority of female uteri. Most American women will die at a ripe old age without ever experiencing problems from their fibroids, or even knowing they had them. Fibroids are usually not a problem, but they can grow to produce extremely bothersome symptoms such as bleeding, pain, or infertility, which can drastically lower a woman's quality of life. The symptoms of fibroids can be troublesome, or even unbearable.

The good news is that many new treatments can control symptoms without surgery. Hysterectomies are often recommended for women with fibroids, but there are many other options.

Hysterectomies do offer women the certainty of an absolute cure for fibroids, but many hysterectomies are unnecessary, the medical equivalent of killing flies with a sledgehammer. Lifestyle strategies, medical therapies, uterine fibroid embolization, and less invasive forms of surgery can help most women control fibroids without undergoing hysterectomy. Many new treatments control symptoms and make life livable again.

Fibroids have a tendency to run in families. Educated women are more likely to get them. For unknown reasons, black women have a much higher incidence of fibroids than white, Hispanic, or Asian women. Women who have never had children are most likely to be diagnosed with fibroids.

Women who are obese or women with diabetes or high blood pressure may be more likely to have a problem with fibroids.

> Fibroids are more common than many women think. One African American woman we know, a college professor at a major university, recalls going to a party with about eight of her women friends. She mentioned in passing that she had fibroids, which had recently been diagnosed.
>
> "I have fibroids," volunteered one friend.
>
> "I have them too," said another.
>
> Altogether, about half the women at the party said they had fibroids. After they talked about them, the college professor no longer felt quite so isolated or alone.

Who Gets Fibroids?

Race	Incidence*	Population of Women**	New Cases Diagnosed Annually
Black	30.6 per 1,000	18,309,891	560,283
White	8.9 per 1,000	98,476,381	876,440
Asian	8.0 per 1,000	5,489,427	43,915
Hispanic	11.0 per 1,000	16,089,357	176,983
American Indian/ Alaskan Native	Not determined	1,201,634	Not determined

Source: National Uterine Fibroids Foundation.

* "Incidence" is the number of *new* diagoses of fibroids made each year for every thousand women, as confirmed by ultrasound or hysterectomy. Incidence statistics source: Marshall LM, Spiegelman D, Barbieri RL, Goldman MB, Manson JE, Colditz GA, Willett WC, Hunter DJ. "Variation in the incidence of uterine leiomyoma among premenopausal women by age and race." *Obstet Gynecol* 1997 Dec;90(6);967-73.

** Population of women source: National Women's Law Center, "Making the Grade on Women's Health 2001."

The uterus supports new life in the form of a developing fetus. While the uterus is not as vital to life as the heart, kidneys, or lungs, it is not a disposable organ. Few men or women want to lose a part of their bodies. The uterus is an important *symbolic* organ for many women, a testament to their femininity and a living witness to their role in carrying on the human race. The uterus may also play a role in a woman's normal hormone balance and be involved in orgasm and sexual response.

Over the ages the uterus has been shrouded in mystery and myth. Some primitive peoples endowed the uterus with magic powers, celebrating it as the very crucible of life. The ancient Egyptians regarded the uterus as a sort of free-roaming animal that moved around a woman's body and acted independently of the woman herself. Over the ages the uterus has been viewed not only as a sexual organ, but also as a source of energy and vitality, and as an organ that helps every woman maintain her youth and attractiveness. Whatever else may be said about it, the uterus is important for the continuation of the human race, the only location on earth in which a fertilized egg can develop into a newborn baby.

Despite the amazing properties of the uterus, many doctors don't think twice about removing it. Beginning in the 1970s physician authors were asserting the limited usefulness of a woman's uterus. In *All about Hysterectomy*, published in 1977, Dr. Harry C. Huneycutt, a Duke University–trained gynecologist, wrote, ". . . the uterus is essentially only a baby carriage. . . ." Dr. Philip Cole, an epidemiologist and head of the

Harvard School of Public Health, wrote in 1979: "If a woman is 35 or 40 years old and has an organ that is disease prone and of little or no further use, it might as well be removed." Are these statements really true?

Imagine a man coming to his doctor's office with a benign tumor on one testicle. His doctor informs him that removing the benign tumor and leaving the testicle gives him more than an 80 percent chance of permanent cure. However, the good doctor confidently recommends surgery to remove both testicles because it will guarantee no recurrence of the tumors.

"We want to take your testicles, but we'll *guarantee* you'll never get another benign tumor," the doctor might tell the frightened man.

"But my testicles are part of me," the patient protests. "These are my body parts, and I'd like to keep them."

While this example may seem absurd, some gynecologists are recommending a similar solution to women: hysterectomies for benign tumors called fibroids. Just remove that little uterus, and you'll get rid of fibroids forever too. Too many times, women are told hysterectomies are "the only reasonable option." Well, times have changed. This is no longer true.

ADVICE AND CONSENT

Many women become confused when they receive the diagnosis of fibroids. Being confused makes them vulnerable, and they are inclined to trust their doctors' advice about fibroids. Unfortunately, many doctors have been trained to believe that when fibroids reach a certain size, the only way to proceed is with a hysterectomy. This is not always the best advice. While this surgery does get rid of the fibroids along with the uterus and generally improves the quality of life for most women who choose it, there *are* many other options. When treating benign conditions such as fibroids, what the *patient* wants is at least as important as what the doctor recommends.

In so frequently recommending hysterectomies for fibroids, some doctors shirk their important advisory and educational role. A good, ethical medical doctor presents *all* medical options to the patient, offers an assessment, and allows the patient to decide. However, some doctors try to push patients toward what the doctor believes is the most reasonable option, even if the patient wants something else. In some cases, recommending a hysterectomy may make sense, but it should still be part of a discussion that includes all appropriate treatment options.

A good doctor explains the risks and benefits of each treatment and helps you choose a treatment that is right for you. Even so, this process takes time, and most doctors do not have much time to spend with patients these days. It's not that doctors are greedy or don't care about their patients; some doctors simply feel it is a waste of time to explain every fibroid treatment option to their patients when a hysterectomy will solve the problem once and for all. Some doctors and patients are uncomfortable with long, emotional conversations about a wide range of medical treatments and troublesome side effects. Many doctors can't answer questions about alternative therapies, vitamin supplements, or other therapies they didn't study in medical school.

This book aims to provide what many doctors can't or won't: unbiased, detailed information on all your treatment options. Armed with this information, you will be able to work together with your doctor to choose the best possible treatment for your situation.

UNNECESSARY SURGERIES

After cesarean delivery, hysterectomy is the most common operation performed on American women. Every ten minutes, twelve hysterectomies are performed in the United States. According to the National Health Interview Survey, uterine fibroids are the most common reason for hysterectomy. Hysterectomy is used much more in the United States than in Europe. Among American women aged eighteen to fifty, more than nine women in every thousand will be advised by their doctors to have a hysterectomy this year. While articles in scientific journals detailing the overuse of hysterectomy date back to the 1940s, there has been essentially no change in hysterectomy rates since that time.

We recently led a government-funded research study that found that perhaps *three-fourths* of all women are undergoing hysterectomies without a thorough medical evaluation. Published in the medical journal *Obstetrics and Gynecology* and conducted under the auspices of the RAND Corporation, we used a panel of medical experts to examine the appropriateness of nearly five hundred hysterectomies done on California women by almost a hundred different Southern California doctors. In an astounding *76 percent* of cases, doctors failed to meet professional treatment criteria set by the American College of Obstetricians and Gynecologists when recommending hysterectomies. Too often, important diagnostic tests, as well as less invasive and more conservative treatments, were skipped as doctor after doctor rushed their female patients onto the fast track for a hysterectomy.

In our study, a surprising *6 percent* of women who had a hysterectomy to treat fibroids *did not even have fibroids* when pathologists carefully examined their uteri after the procedure.

This suggests that tens of thousands of women who have hysterectomies for fibroids do not even have fibroids. As surprising as this sounds, other studies have found the same thing. An analysis published in the *Journal of Public Health* found that 4 to 9 percent of women who underwent hysterectomy for fibroids had *no evidence of fibroids.*

Facts about Fibroids

Here are some facts about fibroids:

- As many as 77 percent of all women have fibroids.
- Between 20 and 40 percent of fibroids create symptoms such as excessive bleeding or pain.
- Over six hundred thousand hysterectomies are performed in the United States each year, 89 percent of them for benign conditions.
- Fibroids account for approximately 45 percent of all hysterectomies.
- Women using hormone replacement therapy are at greater risk for continued symptoms of fibroids compared to women who do not use hormone replacement therapy.

According to our study, many doctors did not perform endometrial biopsies to diagnose the cause of abnormal bleeding, something that is often standard procedure to rule out uterine cancer. Many women with bleeding and pain from their fibroids were never given a chance to see if drug treatments could control their symptoms. In many cases, doctors didn't do enough to rule out other causes of pain before recommending hysterectomy. It is unthinkable that the physicians whose patients we studied intended to harm their patients. However, in three out of every four cases, doctors neglected potentially useful treatments and tests, possibly leading many women to have much more invasive treatment than they needed.

Since 1945 study after study has revealed that *huge* numbers of hysterectomies performed on American women are unnecessary. Although the large majority of women tell their doctors they are doing just fine after a hysterectomy, small but significant numbers of women are psychologically or physically damaged and experience compromised libido, diminished sexual enjoyment, or pain. Unnecessary hysterectomies may contribute to an early and sometimes painful menopause, creating a cascade of overlapping symptoms that can sometimes be countered only by additional medical treatment in the form of hormone replacement therapy.

In our study, fully 14 percent of the women met *no* valid medical criteria for undergoing a hysterectomy. While hysterectomies may have been an appropriate recommendation for some of the women, for at least 14 percent in this study, the recommendation was dead wrong. It is a little frightening to think that so many women undergo major surgery without adequate evaluations, or without the chance to try treatments that might have controlled the symptoms with less risk.

FINANCIAL COSTS

The treatment of fibroids has a huge impact on our health care system. Costs include billions of dollars for conventional and alternative treatments, surgeries, medicines, insurance payments, hospitalization, and days lost from work. In 1997 the U.S. Department of Health and Human Services estimated the costs for surgical and other inpatient care for women with fibroids at more than $2 billion every year, and even this is understated.

Hysterectomy costs an average of approximately $6,000 per surgery, which alone adds up to more than $1 billion per year. Hysterectomies for fibroids cause women to spend nine hundred thousand days in the hospital per year, more days than are spent in the hospital for either breast cancer or AIDS. Myomectomies to remove fibroids cost approximately $5,000 apiece, adding another $200 million per year. When office visits, drugs, and diagnostic procedure costs are included, the cost of treating fibroids easily exceeds $3 billion per year.

If you look at such things as time missed from work, child care, or recovery care costs provided by husbands or other relatives, the amount of time lost to fibroids is staggering. If the average woman with symptoms such as bleeding or pain misses only two days a month from work in the six months before and the six weeks after hysterectomy, then fibroids cause between five and eleven million lost days of work every year.

Risk Factors for Fibroids

- Fibroids develop more commonly in women who began menstruating at younger ages.
- Black women are two to three times more likely than white women to be diagnosed with fibroids.
- Women who have never had children develop fibroids more than women who have.
- Women who have had four to five children are at the lowest risk of all: 70 to 80 percent less likely to develop fibroids than those who have no children. (Miscarriages or abortions do not change the risk of getting fibroids.)
- Obese or overweight women tend to have more problems with fibroids.
- Use of birth control pills has no effect on the development of fibroids.
- Fibroids run in families. One study suggested that women are twice as likely to develop fibroids if they run in the family.
- Women who have gone through menopause are less likely to be diagnosed with fibroids.
- Women who smoke are less likely to develop fibroids (even so, the adverse health effects of smoking far outweigh any possible benefits).

These figures do not even include the money spent on newer treatment alternatives such as uterine fibroid embolization, drug treatments that work, or even alternative therapies. These figures do not include money spent on treatments for related psychological problems such as anxiety and depression, and certainly the emotional costs are incalculable. Despite the phenomenal cost of fibroids, tragically little is spent on researching this condition. The dearth of research into new, less invasive treatments has undoubtedly contributed to doctors' overuse of hysterectomy.

ABOUT THIS BOOK

This book is written for the woman who wants to learn more about fibroids. While not intended as medical advice, this book does include information on tests and new treatments that your doctor may not have the time to explain during a short office visit. This first chapter introduced the topic of fibroids, offered some surprising statistics, and looked at overall costs of treating fibroids.

In the next few chapters we will explain how fibroids grow and develop, look at how doctors diagnose fibroids, discuss the medical tests used, and explain how your doctor can distinguish fibroids from other conditions, such as adenomyosis and ovarian cysts. In addition, we will help you understand the major symptoms of fibroids, including excessive bleeding, pain, sexual issues, and problems with fertility or pregnancy.

In the core of this book we explain why "watchful waiting" may be the best strategy for dealing with fibroids. Diet, exercise, and stress reduction can all help you to control your fibroid symptoms and may reduce the incidence and recurrence of fibroids. We will discuss what you can do about each of these items in taking charge of your own personal health.

In covering your potential treatment options for symptomatic fibroids, we discuss alternative medical treatments such as acupuncture, herbs, and homeopathy as well as conventional drug treatments, which may be useful in controlling your symptoms or shrinking your fibroids.

In the last third of the book we cover uterine fibroid embolization, the most promising and important new technique in the battle against fibroids. Pioneered in the United States by Scott Goodwin, M.D., this book's lead author, uterine fibroid embolization is a safe, reliable alternative to surgery for many women with fibroids. In addition, we examine myomectomy, surgery to remove fibroids without removing the uterus, along with hysterectomy, the most definitive but also the most invasive fibroid treatment.

In closing, we take a brief look at promising but experimental new treatments.

A helpful resources section at the back of the book lists books, professional organizations, and Internet sources of interest. A glossary explains common medical terms.

MOVING AHEAD

You should use this book as a starting point to educate yourself about the newest and best medical treatments for fibroids. No matter what you may have heard from friends. relatives, or doctors, fibroids are harmless most of the time and usually do not need to be removed with a radical operation such as a hysterectomy.

You may be scared by the diagnosis of fibroids, but take heart; there are many good treatments for women with fibroids. More information than ever before is available to the average person, and progress is being made by the day. Many doctors are becoming open to a variety of new approaches to the treatment of fibroids, some of which may be able to reduce or eliminate the need for surgery.

We hope much unnecessary suffering can be prevented as women become more knowledgeable about fibroids, since in an age of continuous medical progress, an educated patient is the best patient of all.

Chapter 2

What Are Fibroids?

More than 99 percent of uterine tumors are not cancerous. This is why they are called *benign* tumors. Fibroids are definitely *not* cancerous. Furthermore, fibroids cannot change into cancerous tumors. The most important thing to understand about fibroids is that they don't usually require treatment unless they cause troublesome symptoms such as bleeding, pain, infertility, urinary problems, or abdominal pressure. Only you can decide what makes symptoms troublesome enough to need treatment.

A slender, athletic registered nurse named Deborah was told she had fibroids nine years ago, when she was thirty-four. Originally, Deborah had gone to see her gynecologist because she thought her belly felt "full" all the time. After a complete examination, Deborah's doctor told her she had thirteen fibroids, one the size of a grapefruit. Deborah was told she should have a hysterectomy, but she resisted.

Some doctors say, "Hey, you're a certain age, you don't need your uterus," Deborah ruefully remembers. "I don't think doctors should tell women that. Psychologically, when I was told I should get a hysterectomy, it just blew me away. The nerve of this person, I thought. I was very upset. I left that doctor's office and never looked back."

She went to another doctor she knew, who explained other treatment options. Deborah ultimately decided to undergo a myomectomy—surgery that removes fibroids but not the uterus. Deborah underwent her first myomectomy seven years ago.

"My uterus was so distorted," she recalls. "I felt if I didn't have surgery, eventually I'd have to have a hysterectomy."

Deborah got along just fine for several years. But several months ago she discovered that her fibroids had grown back. Her periods were nightmares—twenty sanitary pads a night. This monthly loss of blood seriously frightened her and greatly disrupted her life. Not only that, she had become seriously anemic. Her hemoglobin was slightly over 7.0, and her hematocrit was 23, dangerously low.

Deborah found a young doctor affiliated with a local university who had just removed fifty-three fibroids from one of her friends. She trusted this particular doctor, whom she describes as "a cool guy," capable of handling difficult surgeries. When advised of her options, Deborah decided she still did not want a hysterectomy.

To build herself up before the surgery, Deborah worked out in a gym and trained with a personal trainer for three months. She also ran, but at times she got so tired while running she could hardly breathe because of the anemia caused by her fibroids.

In June 2001, at the age of forty-three, Deborah underwent another myomectomy; seventeen fibroids were removed. However, Deborah continued to bleed after the procedure, requiring numerous transfusions, and ultimately underwent uterine artery embolization to control postoperative bleeding. The excessive bleeding was quickly halted.

Today Deborah remains health conscious. She watches her diet, incorporating lots of vegetables and fruits, and works out on a regular basis to keep slim. Looking back, Deborah is happy she was able to avoid what she saw as the worst-case scenario—hysterectomy.

"I saved my body part," says Deborah, who continues to work as a nurse. "If I had had my uterus removed, it would have been like taking a part of me away."

WHAT ARE FIBROIDS?

Fibroids are also called fibroid tumors, uterine fibroids, myomas, leiomyomas, myofibromas, fibromas, fibromyomas, tumors, or benign tumors. Fibroid type tumors may appear many places in the body, including the lungs, but the vast majority grow in the uterus. In one study of women who had had hysterectomies, most for reasons other than fibroids, 74 percent of women before menopause and 84 percent of women after menopause had fibroids. Some experts estimate that as many as *half* of all American women currently have fibroids, but the number may be much higher as most women have no symptoms and therefore don't even realize they have them. Since they are the most common tumors found in the body, it is truly amazing that no one really knows why they develop.

In most women, fibroids don't cause a problem. Studies estimate that between 20 and 50 percent of women diagnosed with fibroids have bothersome symptoms. (The symptoms of fibroids are discussed in chapter 4.)

Fibroids may grow slowly or rapidly. They also sometimes shrink spontaneously. Some fibroids never grow much larger than when they are first detected. Fibroid growth can be tracked accurately with medical tests, but the rate of growth cannot be predicted.

This means that even if fibroids are getting bigger, which they don't always do, no one can say with certainty when, or if, they will grow to any particular size. That is why the advice to "do something now before they get bigger" is usually bad advice. After all, if ten years could go by without any problems, why invite trouble by taking on the risks associated with treatment by having surgery now?

Some fibroids grow like wildfire and keep growing. In exceptional cases, fibroids have gotten very big. The largest fibroid ever reported weighed more than 140 pounds. This is definitely not the norm, as most women have only a few small fibroids. However, in rare cases several hundred have been found in a single woman. For the majority of women, fibroids are manageable without surgery until menopause, when they stabilize or even shrink.

Almost 80 percent of fibroids are diagnosed in women between thirty and fifty years of age, although the range might be considerably more than that. We have had patients as young as twenty-two who have required myomectomies for fibroids and women in their late fifties who are diagnosed with fibroids. On average, black women are diagnosed with fibroids at age thirty-eight, while white women are typically diagnosed at age forty-two.

The vast majority of women with fibroids have more than one. More and more commonly, women are being diagnosed with this condition based on ultrasound and do not have any symptoms at the time they're diagnosed. Pregnancy is a common time to get an ultrasound, and many women with asymptomatic fibroids are diagnosed during this time.

THE AMAZING UTERUS

Fibroids usually form in the wall of the uterus. Positioned just above the vagina and the cervix, and lying deep within the pelvis, the uterus looks a little like a soft, pink, upside-down pear. The uterus is approximately three inches long, and weighs about a quarter of a pound. The inner lining of the uterus is called the *endometrium*. Normally less than a quarter of an inch thick, the endometrium is surrounded by a layer of symmetrically arranged muscle fibers called the *myometrium*, and this is covered by a smooth outer surface called the *serosa*.

The uterus is muscular. Smooth muscle fibers within the uterus are unique since they can stretch out to accommodate a developing baby. Uterine muscles are strong enough to exert 150 pounds of pressure per square inch, the strength necessary to push a baby out of the womb during childbirth. The muscles of the uterus contract every month during menstruation, producing the sometimes painful sensation of cramps.

Fibroids begin growing from a single cell somewhere within the uterine wall. During this process, muscle fibers in the uterus actually change: As cells divide, they become circular masses of tissue that have a whorled appearance under the microscope. This tough fibrous tissue is firm, rather than soft like the typical uterus; this is why a doctor can feel fibroids during a pelvic examination. Usually roughly spherical in shape, a fibroid looks something like a small white or pink potato.

Unlike cancer, fibroids cannot spread. They remain in one location, which makes them harmless to other parts of the body, but fibroids can grow and cause symptoms where they are rooted. As uterine fibroids grow, the arteries supplying them grow as well to assure them an adequate blood supply.

HOW BIG ARE THEY?

The size of fibroids factors into treatment decisions, and doctors describe the size of fibroids in various ways. Some gynecologists describe the size of an enlarged uterus by measuring the volume in cubic centimeters, or by measuring the diameter in centimeters. Your doctor may compare your uterus either to the size of a uterus in a particular stage of pregnancy, or to the size of a common object—fruit and sports seem to be the most popular categories. So a doctor might compare your uterus to a fruit such as an orange or a grapefruit or a ball such as a tennis ball or softball.

Estimating the size of your uterus by describing it in terms of weeks does not mean the fibroid has been growing for that long. This estimation of size compares the entire uterus, including the fibroids, to the size of a typical uterus after so many weeks of pregnancy. If your doctor tells you your uterus is the size of a fourteen-week pregnancy, or the size of a grapefruit, this does not usually mean the fibroid is this size. Your doctor is estimating the size of your *entire* uterus, including the fibroids. Although they are hard, fibroids are not particularly heavy, and they usually are not substantially related to overall weight gain, much to the disappointment of many women with large fibroids. Fibroids that have grown to the size of a twenty-week pregnancy usually weigh only about four or five pounds. It's certainly true, however, that just having fibroids, as well as symptoms from fibroids, can make it hard to exercise or stay active. Of course, reduced activity could certainly contribute to excess weight gain.

Pregnancy Reference	Pelvic Height Reference	Fruit Comparison	Sports Comparison	Inches	Centimeters	Weight*
Normal uterus		Small pear	Tennis ball (2⅞ in.) or hockey puck (3 in.)	3 in.	7.5 cm	8 oz
10 weeks		Orange	Baseball (9 in. in circumference)	3.5 in.	9 cm	12 oz
12 weeks	Just up to the level of the pubic bone	Grapefruit	Softball (12 in. in circumference)	4.5 in.	11.5 cm	1–2 lb
16 weeks	4 finger-breadths above the pubic bone	Melon		6.3 in.	16 cm	~3–5 lb
22 weeks	At the navel	Pineapple	Soccer ball 8⅞ in.	8.7 in.	22 cm	~8–12 lb
28 weeks	3 finger-breadths above the navel	Pumpkin	Football 10⅞ in.	11 in.	28 cm	~17.5–25 lb

Source: National Uterine Fibroids Foundation.

*All weight measurements are approximate calculations based on the measurements identified in this table *and* clinical experience.

Many gynecologists have been taught that a woman needs a hysterectomy when the uterus reaches the size of a large grapefruit, or the size of a twelve-week pregnancy. At that size, the uterus interferes with a doctor's ability to feel enlarged ovaries, and enlarged ovaries may be the first sign of ovarian cancer. With new, more accurate ultrasound and MRI, this argument just doesn't hold up. If a doctor can't feel your ovaries, he or she can simply order one of these tests, which can measure the ovaries more accurately than a pelvic exam.

Doctors give several arguments for performing hysterectomies on women with large fibroids and no symptoms. Women should understand that times have changed, and that each rationale is usually false, as later chapters explain. Even if you have large fibroids, if they don't bother you, or if you can live comfortably with the problems they create, you don't need to take drastic steps to treat them.

TYPES OF FIBROIDS

Fibroids may appear inside, outside, or in the middle of the uterine wall. Doctors use professional jargon to describe their placement in or around the uterus. Remember that what really matters is your symptoms and the treatment your doctor proposes, not the type of fibroids, although the location of fibroids can factor into the type of surgery recommended to remove them. Here is the way doctors classify fibroids:

Subserosal fibroids are the most common type. They grow on the outside of the uterine wall, and they are among the easiest to remove surgically. These can press on the bladder or rectum, organs that are next to the uterus.

Submucosal fibroids are located inside the uterus and under the endometrium. These fibroids grow into the cavity of the uterus, much the same way a baby would develop inside the uterus. Submucosal fibroids may produce heavy or irregular bleeding.

Intramural fibroids are embedded in the middle of the uterine wall. These fibroids can cause the same symptoms as subserosal fibroids and submucosal fibroids, depending on their size and exact location.

Pedunculated fibroids grow on a stalk attached to the uterus, and they make little direct contact with the uterine wall. If the stalk is long, they look a little like a ball on a string. If the stalk is short, they can resemble mushrooms.

A few other forms of fibroids are not located in the uterine wall.

Cervical fibroids, an uncommon type, are located on the cervix or lower segment of the uterus (the part that the doctor examines with a Pap smear).

Intraligamentous fibroids or *broad ligament fibroids* grow directly in the ligaments supporting the uterus, and removal is quite difficult. These types of fibroids often get their blood supply from outside the uterus, possibly making medications and some treatments to shrink fibroids less effective on them.

Intracavitary protruding and *pedunculated submucosal fibroids* protrude into the endometrial cavity and may prevent a successful pregnancy. These fibroids can be removed with a minimally invasive technique called hysteroscopic surgery.

Occasionally a fibroid will develop layers of calcium deposits. These *calcified* fibroids will probably not shrink with medical treatment, but they may stop growing and usually won't get any larger.

FEMALE HORMONES

Much remains to be learned about how fibroids develop. For a long time doctors believed that the hormones estrogen and progesterone regulated fibroid growth. The truth appears to be far more complicated.

Hormones are chemical messengers that trigger effects in parts of the body distant from where the hormones are produced. Estrogen and progesterone, produced in the ovaries, trigger monthly menstrual cycles and have a wide variety of other effects throughout the body. For years doctors thought estrogen was the only important hormone regulator of fibroid growth. Fibroids have many more receptors for estrogen, and therefore bind more estrogen, than the rest of the uterus does. Fibroids convert *estradiol*, the strongest form of estrogen, into *estrone*, a less powerful form, much more slowly than normal uterine tissue. So the local concentration of estrogen, the level in the area just surrounding the fibroid, can be much higher than the level in a nearby part of the uterus.

Although not the whole story, estrogen does play an important role in the appearance of fibroids. Fibroids are uncommon before puberty, they can increase in size during pregnancy, and they usually recede after menopause, all in tandem with rising and falling levels of estrogen in the body. However, if high doses of estrogen caused fibroids, millions of women would have developed fibroids during the 1960s and 1970s, when birth control pills containing estrogen became popular. This didn't happen; birth control pills don't cause fibroids, nor does hormone replacement therapy. Although many dietary and herbal treatments for fibroids attempt to lower estrogen levels, these treatments are not overwhelmingly successful This is most likely because estrogen is not the only hormone to affect fibroid growth.

Fibroids also have receptors for the other major female steroid hormone, progesterone, indicating that progesterone may also have a role in the development of fibroids. Studies have shown that some synthetic progesterone-like substances, called progestins, can increase fibroid size. Some so-called antiprogesterone agents such as mifepristone (also known as the abortion pill, RU-486), which act to block progesterone, can shrink fibroids. These facts lend support to the notion that progesterone also enhances fibroid growth. There is clearly a strong relationship between fibroids and steroid hormones. However, in research to date, manipulating these hormones by taking estrogen or progesterone supplements or by limiting the intake of hormone-rich substances has not been found to predictably affect fibroids.

CANCER AND FIBROIDS

When a woman hears she has a *tumor*, even a benign tumor, her mind jumps immediately to the possibility of cancer. The fear of cancer is intense and real, but it is also a red herring when it is associated with fibroids. Fibroids are *not* cancerous. Furthermore, the chance that a benign tumor such as a fibroid will develop cancer cells is incredibly small. In fact, the chances are very small that *any* solid tumor growing in the wall of the uterus is cancer. By definition, fibroids are *not* malignant, but because cancer can be deadly, your doctor must rule out cancer before proceeding with treatment for fibroids.

One outspoken woman we know went to a different gynecologist every year for her annual examination, looking for one who would remove her fibroids. Despite her excessive bleeding, this woman went for a few years without being checked for cancer. By the time she finally had a test called an endometrial biopsy to look for cancer, she tested positive for endometrial hyperplasia, a cancer precursor. She is furious about this now, since she realizes she should have been given an endometrial biopsy years ago.

Many women have similar experiences. Doctors may choose not to do certain tests for cancer, believing the tests are unnecessary if the patient has the recommended hysterectomy, and a pathologist checks the uterus for cancer after the uterus is removed.

"Gynecologists like this could be giving their patients a death sentence by recommending a hysterectomy and not doing the right tests," this woman says. "In many cases, patients never go back to a particular doctor again because they don't want to have a hysterectomy. When doctors don't perform appropriate diagnostic tests, I'm afraid that some women may not even be aware they are walking out of the office with cancer."

Cancer can develop just about anywhere in the human body, including the breasts, the vagina, the cervix, the endometrium or lining of the uterus, and the ovaries. Heavy bleeding, or bleeding between periods, common reasons that women consult a doctor, can be symptoms of either fibroids *or* cancer. Foul-smelling vaginal discharges can accompany vaginal cancer or cervical cancer. Endometrial cancer can produce spotty bleeding or bleeding between periods. Ovarian cancer can cause bloating or a feeling of a growth in the pelvic area. With the exception of ovarian cancer, these cancers can often be ruled out by tests done in your doctor's office. An ultrasound or MRI can almost always distinguish between uterine fibroids and ovarian cancer.

Rarely, what is first thought to be a fibroid will turn out to be a uterine tumor called a *leiomyosarcoma* or LMS. Fortunately, this type of cancer is extremely rare, affecting less than one in a thousand women who have hysterectomies for fibroids. Leiomyosarcoma occurs in only 0.1 to 0.3 percent of hysterectomies done on women before menopause, and in 1 percent of women having a hysterectomy for fibroids after menopause. This rare malignant tumor affects older women more commonly than younger ones. The average age of women diagnosed with leiomyosarcoma is fifty-eight, about twenty years older than the average age of women treated for symptomatic fibroids.

To test the relationship between this type of cancer and fibroids, Dr. William Parker and several colleagues reviewed the medical records of more than 1,300 women operated on for symptomatic uterine fibroids or "rapidly growing" fibroids. Only three of these women, or less than one-fourth of 1 percent, had a leiomyosarcoma. While many doctors believe that rapid fibroid growth is a sign of cancer, of the 370 women operated on because their fibroids were growing rapidly in this study, only one had a cancer. This study concluded that there is "no justification for assuming that growth in a fibroid means that cancer is developing." The study's authors recommend that women with rapidly growing fibroids have frequent pelvic examinations, but they do not need surgery simply because the fibroids are growing.

In 1999 a second study looked at the records of almost one thousand women at one hospital, ages thirty-nine to fifty, who had had hysterectomies for fibroids. Only one case of leiomyosarcoma was found, which translates to 0.1 percent of the population studied.

Of the other types of cancer that can occur in the female genital tract, most are easy to detect, easy to control, or statistically rare.

Cervical cancer is usually a very slow growing cancer. Women who go to the doctor for regular Pap smears do not usually develop cervical cancer. Pap smears usually detect cervical cancer in the precancerous state, called *cervical dysplasia*, and dysplasia is easily treated without major surgery by using freezing or heat to remove the abnormal cells. Cervical dysplasia occurs most often in women in their twenties and thirties, and it can take twenty years for cervical dysplasia to develop into cancer. If a Pap smear shows dysplasia, a biopsy can rule out cervical cancer.

Endometrial cancer, also called *endometrial carcinoma*, develops in the lining of the uterus and accounts for an estimated 13 percent of all cancers in women. However, it is the least deadly of the female cancers, with a cure rate of more than 90 percent if detected in its early stages. The precancerous stage, which is *not* yet cancer, is called *endometrial hyperplasia*. This stage often causes abnormal bleeding, as does endometrial cancer. Bleeding between periods can be a symptom of endometrial cancer, particularly if you are over thirty-five. Your doctor should rule this out with ultrasound or endometrial biopsy before treating your fibroids. When properly treated, endometrial hyperplasia rarely progresses to cancer.

Endometrial cancer and hyperplasia both result from an excess of circulating estrogen. Most cases of endometrial hyperplasia will go away on their own or with hormone treatment. Some specific types of hyperplasia are more likely to go away than others will; your doctor can determine the type with an endometrial biopsy. Because fat cells produce estrogen, overweight women are at greater risk of endometrial hyperplasia and endometrial cancer, as they have higher levels of circulating estrogen in their bloodstream. Women who have never had children; have high blood pressure or diabetes; or experience early onset of menstruation, irregular periods, or a late menopause are statistically at a greater risk for endometrial hyperplasia. Treatment for both hyperplasia and early endometrial cancer involves either taking hormones to counter estrogen's effects, or hysterectomy. Unless the cancer is very advanced and is spread outside the uterus, even later stages of endometrial carcinoma are completely cured by a hysterectomy.

Ovarian cancer affects about one in eighty women. The median age for ovarian cancer is fifty-nine. The sixth most common cancer among women, it usually occurs after menopause in women between fifty-five and sixty-four, but sometimes affects younger women too. Ovarian cancer can be quite deadly.

Ovarian cancer has a higher cure rate when it is discovered in the early stages, but since the ovaries are buried in the abdominal cavity, most ovarian cancers are not found until they are fairly advanced. A CA-125 "tumor marker" blood test is sometimes used to help diagnose ovarian cancer. Unfortunately, fibroids and other benign conditions can raise the level of CA-125 even though no cancer is present.

Most ovarian cancer is detected after the cancer has spread, when it is rarely curable. Other than a thorough examination and perhaps an ultrasound, there is nothing a doctor can or should routinely do to try to rule out ovarian cancer. Even having a hysterectomy does not prevent ovarian cancer since it can occur even after the uterus and ovaries have been removed. This strange situation is called *primary peritoneal cancer* and happens because microscopic areas of ovarian cancer can begin outside the ovaries themselves, on the thin layer of cells, the peritoneum, that lines the pelvis.

Vaginal cancer is extremely rare, mostly occurring in women who have been exposed to diethylstilbestrol or DES, a synthetic estrogen once given to pregnant women to prevent miscarriage.

The bottom line is that fibroids are not cancer, they don't cause cancer; and they do not even increase the risk of having cancer. They are benign growths that appear in the female uterus and can cause a range of symptoms. Fibroids are classified by size and by location, and both of these factors can affect treatment decisions. By far the most important factor to consider when treating fibroids is whether they are causing symptoms. If not, no treatment is the best treatment.

Cancer

Each year the American Cancer Society (ACS) produces an annual report that forecasts the estimated number of new cancer cases diagnosed as well as the number of deaths expected to occur. Their estimates are based on information obtained from the National Center for Health Statistics at the Centers for Disease Control and Prevention. To place the dangers from the more than one hundred types of cancer potentially affecting women in perspective, the following table shows projected statistical estimates from the ACS 2002 report regarding new cases of cancer expected to be diagnosed in more than one hundred million women in the United States. Combining all cancers, including cancers not identified in the table, 647,400 cases of cancer are anticipated to be diagnosed in women in 2002.

Cancer Site	Estimated New Cases in 2002	Estimated Deaths in 2002
Lung	79,200	65,700
Breast	203,500	39,600
Colon	57,300	25,000
Pancreatic	15,600	15,200
Ovarian	23,300	13,900
Lymphoma	29,000	12,300
Leukemia	13,200	9,600
Uterus*	39,000	6,600
Cervical	13,000	4,100
Urinary bladder	15,000	4,000
Skin	25,800	3,400
Vulvar	3,800	800
Vaginal and all other genital cancers	2,000	800

*Includes endometrial cancer and leiomyosarcoma, which make up a small minority of these cases.

Diagnosing Fibroids

To get the best possible medical care, it is important to form a partnership with your doctor. Communication is a two-way street. Before you can expect your physician to know how to advise you, you must share your concerns.

In the beginning your doctor should take a careful history of your symptoms and any other medical problems you might have, perform a thorough physical examination, and complete a number of tests. Since these tests provide valuable information on your physical condition, each of them has been outlined in this chapter. Depending on your symptoms, your doctor may also try to rule out other conditions sometimes mistaken for fibroids, including adenomyosis, endometriosis, ovarian cysts, and uterine polyps. The better you understand the process of ruling out other diseases to arrive at a diagnosis of fibroids, the better able you will be to work with your doctor to choose your treatment.

A QUESTION OF TRUST

Ultimately, the doctor–patient relationship must be based on trust. The patient must honestly and frankly explain her medical problem and describe her symptoms. The doctor must listen to the patient, ask questions, do a physical examination, order diagnostic tests, and evaluate all the information. Your doctor must eliminate conditions other than fibroids before recommending treatment. In the end, you must approve any treatment for fibroids your doctor recommends.

Most doctors are not psychologists, although many are sympathetic listeners. For better or worse, medical doctors are trained to see the physical disease and not necessarily the human side of the person. This can create a professional distance, preventing them from seeing what would be best for you as an individual, rather than just as a woman with fibroids. Doctors can be brusque, but a bad bedside manner doesn't mean that your doctor is incompetent. You don't have to like your medical doctor, but you should respect his or her medical judgment. However, if the interpersonal relationship you have with your physician is poor enough, it can prevent communication necessary to your medical care. Doctors are experts in how the human body operates, and they should be able to answer any questions you have about your medical condition. If your doctor won't answer your questions to your satisfaction, or rushes you toward a hysterectomy right away, get a second opinion, or a different doctor. You have a right to understand what your doctor is suggesting. If he or she can't or won't help you reach this understanding, find the door.

"My doctor seems to really know what he's doing," says a woman in her early forties who is being treated for fibroids. "He's never talked to me as if I didn't know anything. He gives me the benefit of the doubt that I understand what is going on with my own body. He's not formal, and he's not condescending. I think he's great."

However, a second woman we know was not happy with her gynecologist, a man who spent their entire first appointment trying to talk her into having a hysterectomy. As she left the office, this doctor gave her a feel-good video, which she noticed was sponsored by drug companies involved in hormone replacement therapy, and a comic book full of smiling women talking about how great they felt after having a hysterectomy. These simple-minded educational tools insulted this woman's intelligence and made her feel she was being treated like a child.

To cap it all off, the same gynecologist scheduled her for a hysterectomy without her permission. The woman only found out when the hospital called her to confirm the date of her surgery. She became furious.

"I felt this man had violated my personal dignity and a lot of my rights by scheduling a hysterectomy without my permission," she said. "This was the most horrific interaction I've ever had with a doctor."

She angrily canceled the hysterectomy. The doctor sheepishly called her back and said he'd try to do an operation to remove only her fibroids if she really wanted, but the trust was broken, and our friend began looking for another doctor.

> A third woman recalls: "After my first appointment I knew I'd found the right doctor. He was very professional, and very thorough. He explained everything to me and made the whole thing as painless as possible. I've been very pleased with the level of care I've received." She especially liked the fact that her doctor took the time to explain her treatment options, answered her questions, and followed through after she had decided on a treatment option.

Doctors are trained to listen to your medical concerns and explain a rationale for treatment. If something puzzles you, ask your doctor about it. Here are a few general tips on communicating with your medical doctor:

- Answer all your doctor's questions as frankly as you can. Be prepared to answer questions about symptoms such as the frequency of your bleeding or the extent of menstrual pain.
- Don't be afraid to ask your own questions, or to ask that an answer be repeated if you didn't understand it the first time. Focus questions on your health problems.
- If it will help, prepare a list of questions in advance and give the doctor a copy of your list before you begin. Don't overdo this. If you have more than five or six questions, get the list to the doctor prior to your visit and ask for extra time to have all your questions answered.
- If you have trouble remembering what your doctor says and he or she feels comfortable with it, tape-record your doctor's remarks. Bring a friend or a spouse into a consultation if that helps you remember.
- Ask about the risks and benefits of any treatment suggested.

- If your doctor doesn't answer your questions to your satisfaction, consult another doctor.

MEDICAL TESTS

Before treating you for fibroids, your doctor must be reasonably sure that you actually have them. What doctors call the "workup" consists of a medical history, a physical exam, and tests that can identify or rule out other conditions. Obviously, it's important to get an accurate diagnosis before treatment begins.

Since there is no single right way to diagnose fibroids, different doctors may order different tests. As a way of keeping yourself completely informed, you may want to ask for copies of all test results and keep them in a file for future reference, or to use if you change doctors. Tests that you may encounter include the following:

- Complete blood count (also called a CBC)
- Bimanual examination (or pelvic exam)
- Pap smear
- Ultrasound (also called sonography)
- MRI (magnetic resonance imaging)
- X rays
- Endometrial biopsy (EMB)
- Dilation and curettage (D&C)
- Hysteroscopy
- Laparoscopy

A *complete blood count*, or CBC, is often one of the first things a doctor will order if you have heavy bleeding. Among other things, a CBC detects anemia, a potentially dangerous condition that results from excessive bleeding.

A *bimanual examination*, conducted with both hands, is part of a standard pelvic exam. During this examination, your gynecologist inserts two fingers into your vagina, places the other hand on your stomach, and then gently pushes the cervix and uterus up close to the surface of your skin, where the shape, size, and firmness of the uterus may be felt. Perhaps 90 percent of the time, a doctor finds fibroids this way. An empty bladder is necessary for this exam. Since the bladder is adjacent to the uterus, a full bladder may give your doctor a false idea of uterine size, in addition to making the exam extremely uncomfortable. If your doctor finds that your uterus is enlarged, firm, or has an irregular shape, he or she may suspect that you have uterine fibroids. Because gynecologists are trained in anatomy, they can easily feel if the shape of the uterus is distorted, or if uterine tissue is harder than normal. To the doctor, a uterus with fibroids often feels firm rather than soft. The uterus may feel somewhat enlarged or irregular in shape, as if it has bumps or protrusions. If fibroids are near the outer wall of the uterus, the doctor can easily feel them. If your fibroids are large, you may be able to feel them yourself.

The bimanual examination does not complete a diagnosis of fibroids. Pain, muscular tension, or fat deposits can interfere with a bimanual examination, making a definitive diagnosis more difficult. Other firm masses in the abdomen such as ovarian cysts or even a tilted uterus can be mistaken for fibroids during a bimanual examination. A definitive diagnosis of fibroids usually requires more sophisticated tests. Ultrasound and magnetic resonance imaging are often used for this purpose. Both tests also check the ovaries and can help distinguish fibroids from ovarian masses.

The Pap smear is a common test that has been used since the 1940s to diagnose cervical cancer. Many women misunderstand the use of a Pap smear and believe that it can accurately diagnose all kinds of female cancers. Unfortunately, this isn't the case. It is extremely good at finding early cervical cancer and cervical precancer. The vast majority of women who get Pap smears never die of cervical cancer because their cancers are found very early and are treated appropriately. However, Pap smears cannot diagnose ovarian cancer or many cancers of the uterus. Tests to diagnose uterine cancer, such as the endometrial biopsy, are discussed in more detail later. Although it's hard to mistake cervical cancer for uterine fibroids, it is important that your doctor rule out any abnormalities of the cervix before recommending treatment for your fibroids. For this reason, it's good to make sure you've had a Pap smear in the last year before undertaking any treatment for fibroids.

Ultrasound or *ultrasonography* is the most common and least expensive imaging test for fibroids. Ultrasound can be done quickly, often right in your doctor's office, and is usually painless. Ultrasound devices send inaudible sound waves into the body, which bounce back off the organs, creating "pictures" that give an ultrasound technician or your doctor a somewhat accurate idea of the number and size of your fibroids. Ultrasound scans sometimes need to be done with a full bladder.

An ultrasound report usually indicates how many fibroids are present, their location, and their size. Fibroids will not be identified in this way if many small fibroids are present, in which case a range of sizes is usually given.

During an ultrasound, sound waves are directed either across the abdomen or through the vagina. In *transabdominal* ultrasound, the doctor moves a transducer over your abdomen.

For this test, the bladder should be full. *Transvaginal* scanning involves a lubricated plastic probe inserted into the vagina. Transvaginal ultrasound is more accurate and doesn't require a full bladder. In addition to helping diagnose fibroids, ultrasound can be used to monitor the growth or shrinkage of fibroids during periods of watchful waiting, or to assess fibroids after treatments have begun.

Ultrasound has its limits. A retroverted uterus, one that is tilted back on itself, can appear to be a fibroid on ultrasound. Very small fibroids (less than one centimeter in diameter) often escape detection. If more than five fibroids are present, it can be difficult to differentiate among them using only ultrasound. It is also sometimes difficult to distinguish multiple small fibroids from conditions such as adenomyosis with ultrasound.

The *hysterosonogram*, also called *saline infusion ultrasonography*, involves the injection of a small amount of saltwater into the uterus, followed by a vaginal probe ultrasound. This test helps the doctor distinguish between fibroids and uterine polyps, both of which can cause heavy or irregular bleeding. Saline ultrasound also delineates the endometrial lining and can sometimes rule out endometrial cancer as a cause of bleeding.

MRI or *magnetic resonance imaging* is the most accurate test for fibroids, but it is also more expensive, time-consuming, and can be a little scary. Some doctors routinely use MRI to diagnose fibroids, as this is the most accurate test available. However, simpler and less expensive tests often give nearly as much information. An MRI exam takes place in a special chamber where earplugs protect you from the very loud sounds created by the machine. Most MRI machines are shaped like long tubes, and your whole body goes inside the tube for this exam. MRI is not particularly pleasant for some people since you are stuck in a tight space with loud noises being made close to your ears. Some models of MRI equipment are "open" and do not require the body to move through an enclosed tube to complete the necessary imaging. If an MRI is recommended and you are claustrophobic, be certain to let your doctor know, since this test could be terrifying for a claustrophobic person unless an open MRI is used.

MRI exams do provide an extremely detailed picture of the inside of the body and precisely differentiate fibroids from other tissues. MRI results tell your doctor if fibroids are located deep within the uterine wall or closer to the surface. An MRI is one of the few tests that can differentiate fibroids from adenomyosis.

In addition to tests used to diagnose fibroids, other tests are employed to rule out cancer and other conditions. The simplest of these, an *endometrial biopsy* (EMB) can be done in the doctor's office using a small sampling device that looks a little like a plastic soda straw. To perform an endometrial biopsy, the doctor introduces this thin straw through the cervix. This requires you to be on the exam table, in stirrups, like for a Pap smear. A small amount of suction pulls some cells from the uterine lining into the straw. These sample cells allow a pathologist to determine if cancerous or precancerous changes have occurred in the endometrial lining.

Many women with irregular bleeding should also have an EMB to rule out endometrial cancer as a cause of the bleeding. Endometrial cancer is an uncommon cause of bleeding in women with fibroids, but because this cancer is easy to diagnose, an EMB should be done in certain situations. Endometrial cancer is more common in women who have higher estrogen levels or lower progesterone levels, particularly when higher or lower hormone levels occur for a long period of time.

Women who have regular menstrual periods have a high level of progesterone in the second half of the cycle. This progesterone is produced by the ovulatory follicle that remains after ovulation occurs. Women who don't ovulate regularly (or at all) have lower levels of progesterone, and this puts them at higher risk of endometrial cancer. Women who have had anovulation for long periods of time are at even higher risk.

Because endometrial cancer takes time to develop, it is rarely diagnosed in women under age thirty-five. If you're younger than thirty-five, your doctor may not want to perform this test even if you have had irregular bleeding for many years. Endometrial cancer seldom causes bleeding at regular intervals, so if your periods are heavy but come always at the expected time, this test might not be necessary. In general, performing an EMB on any woman over thirty-five who has bleeding between periods is good medical practice.

An endometrial biopsy is an excellent method of finding endometrial cancer, but some doctors still prefer the older method of dilatation and curettage (D&C), which requires larger instruments and is typically performed in an operating room. D&C is usually done with general anesthesia and may have more procedural risks than endometrial biopsy, but it does provide a slightly higher quantity of tissue for the pathologist to examine. During a D&C, your doctor may also be able to "feel" the lining of the uterus and gain a sense of whether fibroids are protruding into this lining. A D&C can also be useful to remove uterine polyps, which are small fleshy projections inside the cavity of the uterus that can sometimes cause bleeding. Endometrial biopsy is really only a diagnostic test and does not treat heavy bleeding at all.

Hysteroscopy, typically done under a general anesthetic, uses a small, lighted telescope-like device called a *hysteroscope* to view the inside of the uterus. This allows the physician to see and obtain a sample from the area of the uterus that may be responsible for heavy bleeding. In addition, it also allows the doctor to see any small fibroids inside the uterus. Other conditions, which may cause symptoms similar to fibroid-related symptoms, such as uterine polyps or endometrial cancer, may be ruled out with hysteroscopy and D&C. Hysteroscopy can sometimes be used to remove small submucosal fibroids altogether.

Diagnostic laparoscopy is only rarely needed to diagnose fibroids. Laparoscopic surgery involves the insertion of a small tube containing a telescope-like device into the abdomen. A diagnostic laparoscopy can identify very small fibroids in locations such as the outside of the uterus, where they may be hard to see on ultrasound. A laparoscopy can definitively identify *endometriosis*, the second most common female disorder after fibroids. If both fibroids and endometriosis are present, medical treatment can be different than for fibroids alone. Laparoscopic myomectomy, surgery to remove fibroids, is discussed in detail in later chapters.

Some physicians perform a *needle biopsy* of tumors during a diagnostic laparoscopy. This procedure involves inserting small needles into the fibroid tumors and removing samples of tissue for a pathologist to examine under a microscope. The goal of performing a needle biopsy is to rule out the possibility that a uterine fibroid is actually a leiomyosarcoma (LMS), or cancerous tumor. Unfortunately, since LMS is an extremely rare cancer and may actually develop from single cells in any location in the uterus, extracting tissue samples in this manner may miss cancerous cells altogether, should they exist. More important, however, when many tumors are growing in the uterus, it is literally impossible to sample every tumor. For this reason, needle biopsies taken to rule out LMS are an expensive, invasive, and impractical method for diagnosing uterine LMS. Further research is underway, however, which may someday provide improved diagnostic techniques along with even greater assurances of the diagnosis of benign uterine fibroids.

X-ray exams are usually not necessary to diagnose fibroids, but they can pinpoint fibroids that have become calcified. An *intravenous pyelogram*, or IVP, shows the kidneys, ureters, and bladder. The IVP can show a large fibroid pressing against the *ureters*, thin tubes that carry urine from the kidneys to the bladder. This type of pressure has the potential to cause kidney damage if left untreated. An IVP sometimes turns up other rare problems such as abnormally placed kidneys.

After ordering and reviewing these tests, your doctor should have a good picture of your condition. Questions you may want to ask your doctor at this point include the following:

- How many fibroids do I have, and how big are they?
- Have you already ruled out the possibility of cervical or endometrial cancer? (Remember, there are no good tests to rule out early ovarian cancer.)
- What should I do now?
- What treatments might I need in the future, and what are their risks and benefits?

SIMILAR CONDITIONS

Adenomyosis, endometriosis, ovarian cysts, and uterine polyps are all conditions with symptoms that may be similar to the symptoms of fibroids. Adenomyosis, for instance, occasionally causes bleeding or pain and can enlarge the uterus. Endometriosis is hard to confuse with fibroids, but both can cause pain, particularly during menstrual periods. Ovarian cysts usually have no symptoms, but occasionally rupture and cause pain during the middle of the menstrual cycle. Uterine polyps can cause bleeding and pain. These conditions are not fibroids, but when they are present along with fibroids, they can make finding the right diagnosis and choosing a treatment more complex.

• *Adenomyosis*—This condition is commonly mistaken for fibroids since it presents with similar symptoms. Adenomyosis occurs in about 10 percent of women with fibroids. Women in their forties and fifties who have had children are most prone to this condition. Sometimes called "internal endometriosis," adenomyosis can cause severe cramping, pain, and heavy bleeding during periods. Adenomyosis occurs when the lining of the uterus grows directly into the muscle wall. The uterine lining bleeds during menstrual periods, and since this bleeding is somewhat "trapped" in the uterine wall, the uterine muscle swells up, causing pain. To the doctor, adenomyosis feels wooden and fibrous, like a fibroid, during a bimanual examination. To add to the confusion, adenomyosis can be mistaken for fibroids on ultrasound.

Surgery was once the only definitive way to differentiate this condition from fibroids since tissue could be examined under a microscope. These days adenomyosis can also be diagnosed with an MRI or with specialized ultrasound techniques. Treatment is similar to treatment for fibroids—first using medications, then more invasive techniques if the medications fail. Uterine fibroid embolization may show some promise as a treatment for adenomyosis. Surgery may be employed as a last resort, and hysterectomy is usually the surgery of choice. Adenomyosis is usually found spread throughout the uterus, not in discrete tumors like fibroids, making removing just the "abnormal" parts of the uterus difficult.

• *Endometriosis*— Endometriosis occurs when the uterine lining (endometrium), the part of the uterus normally lost during menstruation each month, grows in areas outside the uterus. These *islets of endometrium* can grow on the outside of the uterus, on the ligaments that hold the uterus in place, on the ovaries, on the fallopian tubes, or even as far away as the lungs. During menstruation, these cells begin to bleed, exactly what normal endometrial cells should do, but the blood is not in a normal location inside the uterus.

Painful periods, chronic pain in the pelvis, pain during or after sex (especially during deep penetration), painful bowel movements, sudden pelvic pain, or fertility problems can all be symptoms of endometriosis. Although severe pain during periods can suggest the diagnosis of endometriosis, a biopsy of these endometriotic cells is required to be sure. These biopsies are done using laparoscopy, a technique explained in detail in chapter 12. Treatments for endometriosis involve reducing hormone stimulation of endometrial tissue, which can be accomplished with birth control pills or using hormones similar to progesterone. Stronger drugs, such as Danazol or GnRH agonists (described in chapter 10), can also be effective against the pain of endometriosis. Surgery can usually remove most of the endometriosis and scar tissue, but a combination of medications and surgery often works best. In extreme cases, hysterectomy with removal of ovaries and fallopian tubes may be required to relieve the symptoms. Endometriosis goes away after menopause, when circulating levels of estrogen drop dramatically. Pregnancy improves endometriosis, sometimes even causing permanent relief of symptoms.

• *Ovarian cysts*—A cyst is nothing more than a thin shell

of tissue that contains fluid. Cysts are normal findings in the ovaries of a woman who is ovulating and having periods. The cyst is produced by the egg released from the ovary during ovulation. After the egg is released, the area that produced the egg continues to make a hormone-rich fluid. This resulting ovarian cyst is the source of the progesterone that predominates in the second half of a menstrual cycle. Normally, two weeks after ovulation, the cyst collapses and disappears. This usually coincides with the onset of the menstrual period. For some reason, in some cases the cyst doesn't collapse but rather continues to produce fluid and can enlarge. Because cysts are normally produced in the second half of every menstrual cycle, ultrasounds done to detect fibroids often find coexisting ovarian cysts. Except in unusual cases, these cysts are nothing to be concerned about and do not require any treatment or even further observation. In some cases, particularly if the cysts are large, perhaps more than a few inches across, or have an unusual appearance on ultrasound, they should be investigated further. Usually, further investigation just means repeating ultrasounds later in the month or in a different month. For cysts that don't resolve over time, laparoscopy is sometimes required to determine exactly what is causing them.

• *Uterine polyps*—Uterine or endometrial polyps are small, soft growths that occur inside the uterus. They arise from the lining of the uterus and contain cells that are very similar to normal endometrial cells. These polyps are not cancerous, but they can be mistaken for fibroids, particularly fibroids located inside the cavity of the uterus, called submucosal fibroids. Both polyps and fibroids located inside the uterus can cause abnormal bleeding, perhaps by irritating the normal uterine lining. Both submucosal fibroids and polyps can be diagnosed using saline ultrasound in which a small amount of fluid is injected into the uterus while ultrasound waves are bounced off the uterus in order to create a picture of it and its contents. Polyps and submucosal fibroids can often easily be removed using hysteroscopy (described in chapter 12).

Second Opinions

A few insurance companies require second opinions if major surgery is recommended, although this is less common than a few years ago. Getting a second opinion may also make you feel better about the choices you have for treating fibroids, although you may have to pay for the visit yourself. Getting a second opinion may not change your diagnosis, but it could help you further assess which treatments are most suitable for you.

If you have trouble communicating with your doctor, if you are not confident in his or her judgment, or if you are uncomfortable with what is recommended, think about seeking a second opinion. You may also want to get a second opinion to confirm your doctor's diagnosis and recommendations if your doctor isn't experienced in treating fibroids, or for reassurance that you are getting the most current treatment recommendations available. Be sure to take copies of your records and test results with you to the second consultation. Remember, you would probably get two quotes for any home remodeling work—you should take at least as much care with your body!

Your insurance policy may limit your choice of doctors for a second opinion. Hopefully, your second opinion physician won't be a partner or a close friend of your initial doctor. If you can, pick a doctor who is not affiliated with your doctor. You may want to consult a gynecologist at a nearby university medical center, where doctors are often up on the latest research and treatment techniques. Professional organizations such as the American Medical Association, the American College of Obstetricians and Gynecologists, and the Society of Interventional Radiology often maintain listings of board-certified physicians and list their specialty areas.

If possible, take copies of your records and charts with you to the second consultation, rather than having your doctor's office mail or fax them.

Try to work with your doctor as a partner. Ask your doctor the questions you need to ask, and insist on comprehensible answers. Your doctor should be a trusted advisor and teacher who understands your medical condition and who can explain the rationale for treatment. Understand the tests used to diagnose your fibroids; consider keeping copies of test results. Make sure your physician has ruled out conditions that may be mistaken for fibroids such as adenomyosis, ovarian cysts, and polyps. Only when the diagnostic process is complete are you ready to consider treatment options. As explained in the following chapter, if you have troublesome symptoms that interfere with your life, you may need treatment for fibroids; if you have no symptoms, you probably only need a firm diagnosis and a plan for watchful waiting.

Chapter 4

Managing Symptoms

Fibroids only cause symptoms or noticeable problems in 30 to 50 percent of women who have them, but these symptoms may be bothersome or even, in extreme cases, life threatening. Symptoms may include bleeding, pain, pressure, bloating or feelings of fullness, sexual problems, infertility, and complications during pregnancy. The severity of your symptoms may have a direct impact on the treatments you select for fibroids. The more severe your symptoms are, the more likely you will be to choose invasive treatment.

A thirty-four-year-old computer programmer named Tanya was diagnosed with fibroids six years ago, before she and her husband were thinking of having a child. After a bimanual exam and ultrasound, Tanya was told she had fibroids. Tanya had never even heard of fibroids before. The ultrasound technician told her that she had three good-sized fibroids, one the size of a grapefruit and the others the size of small oranges.

She said, "That seems large. Will I be able to get pregnant?"

"It's not a problem. Lots of women with fibroids have babies," the ultrasound technician said.

A year or so later, however, when Tanya and her husband began trying to have a child, she didn't get pregnant. Thanks to fibroids, Tanya was also experiencing stress incontinence, painful menstrual cramping, and painful intercourse, and these symptoms were affecting her quality of life. She had also begun to gain weight, something no one enjoys. Finally, a doctor of reproductive medicine told Tanya that she could get pregnant, but that her fibroids had become so big that she probably wouldn't carry the baby to term.

Tanya found a good gynecologist. After weighing her treatment choices, she opted for an abdominal myomectomy—surgery that removes the fibroids but leaves the uterus intact.

"After the surgery, I started seeing changes in my body. My incontinence disappeared. My shape changed. I was able to put on a pair of pants I hadn't worn in two years. That does a lot for your whole state of mind," Tanya said.

About a month after the surgery, Tanya was almost back to normal. With the fibroids removed, Tanya and her husband began trying to have a child again.

SYMPTOMS OF FIBROIDS

Several major physical problems or symptoms are associated with uterine fibroids; these symptoms can occur alone or in clusters. Symptoms of fibroids include the following:

- Bleeding
  — Increased menstrual bleeding
  — Bleeding between menstrual periods
- Pain
- Pressure
- Bloating/feeling of fullness
  — Pelvic pressure or a sense of bulkiness
  — The ability to manually feel the fibroid mass in your abdomen
- Sexual dysfunction
  — Pain during or after intercourse
- Infertility
  — Size and/or location of fibroids preventing pregnancy
  — Inflammation preventing pregnancy
- Pregnancy complications
  — Pain
  — Preterm labor
  — Cesarean delivery
- Urinary problems
  — Frequent urination
  — Leaking urine
- Depression

BLEEDING

Some women with fibroids have such severe bleeding that they can't leave the house for several days a month, not even to go to work or to go grocery shopping. Other women bleed so profusely that they must change pads and tampons every hour. This type of bleeding can be embarrassing and humiliating, and it can devastate one's ability to lead a normal life. Bleeding is one of the most common reasons women see a gynecologist, and it can become worse if no steps are taken to control it.

As a rule of thumb, if your periods come more frequently than every twenty-one days, if they last more than seven or eight days, if you bleed between periods, or if your periods suddenly become heavier than they have ever been, you should consult a gynecologist. One instance of abnormal bleeding like this is usually nothing to worry about, but if it happens every month, see your doctor. Excessive menstrual bleeding can cause anemia, weakness, and dizziness. Some studies estimate that 30 percent of women with fibroids have excessive or abnormal bleeding.

Possible Causes of Abnormal Bleeding with Fibroids

- Fibroid tumor growth into the uterine cavity interferes with normal menstrual function
- Blood-clotting mechanisms and normal uterine contractions (which work to stop normal menstrual bleeding) blocked by fibroids
- More blood vessels bringing more blood to uterus
- Uterine congestion caused by fibroids interfering with normal blood flow in and out of the uterus

Doctors can't say with any certainty why fibroids cause excessive bleeding since fibroids themselves don't really bleed, but this is still the most common symptom of fibroids. Although fibroids in any location may potentially cause bleeding, in one recent study, women with intramural or submucosal fibroids were most likely to experience abnormal bleeding.

Fibroids that grow into the uterine cavity (submucosal fibroids) may cause bleeding by interfering with the normal actions of the body. Usually, the body's blood-clotting mechanisms combined with muscular uterine contractions work to stop normal menstrual bleeding. Since fibroids are solid tumors, they may stop the smooth muscles of the uterus from contracting completely.

As fibroids grow, they induce blood vessels to grow and bring more blood to the uterus. Thus, the entire uterus is now receiving more blood than usual. This may explain the heavy bleeding some women experience. Heavy bleeding may also occur because fibroids cause congestion of the uterus with blood by not allowing normal blood flow back to the heart. In other words, the fibroids block the veins that allow blood to flow out of the uterus, and this congestion may lead to heavy bleeding.

Two common patterns of abnormal bleeding occur in women with fibroids. One is longer periods, which is referred to as *menorrhagia* from the Greek words for menstrual period (*meno*) and "to burst forth" (*rrhagia*). Bleeding between periods is called *metrorrhagia* (*metro* means "crowded together"). Some women experience *menometrorrhagia*, in which periods are very heavy and close together. A related medical term, *dysmenorrhea*, refers to pain during menstrual periods. Whereas average women might menstruate four to seven days per month, women with fibroids sometimes have periods lasting eight days or longer. There are also potentially serious health consequences to prolonged, excessive bleeding.

Although it's hard to measure accurately the amount of blood lost during a menstrual period, heavy bleeding does result in a loss of the iron carried in red blood cells, as well as in a loss of other vital nutrients. During an average period, most women lose about two tablespoons of blood. If you lose more than five or six tablespoons of blood per cycle, anemia may result. Anemia means that there are not enough red blood cells circulating. Since red blood cells carry oxygen, there may not be enough oxygen getting to vital organs. Two common tests for anemia are the hematocrit and the hemoglobin test. Normal values can vary a little among laboratories, but are usually 34–42 for hematocrit and 10–14 for hemoglobin.

Anemia

Doctors have two types of tests for anemia. A test for hemoglobin measures the concentration of the oxygen-carrying molecule in the body—normally around twelve to fourteen grams per deciliter of blood. A test of hematocrit measures the percent of the blood that consists of red blood cells, normally around 40 percent.

The following table shows the medical parameters for anemia after a standard blood test. Anemia is a potentially dangerous medical condition often caused by excessive bleeding. These numbers are not set in stone, and can vary from laboratory to laboratory, depending on who is giving and interpreting the test.

Hematocrit	Hemoglobin	Diagnosis
34–42%	12–14 g/dl	Normal
30–33%	10–12 g/dl	Mild anemia
<30%	<10 g/dl	Moderate to severe anemia

Anemia can produce shortness of breath, weakness, fatigue, dizziness, light-headedness, ringing in the ears, and headaches.

These symptoms, all the result of insufficient oxygen in the brain, can be a warning sign of even worse problems such as heart attack or heart failure. Iron supplements are commonly prescribed for anemia to replace the lost iron the body needs to build new red blood cells. Iron supplements can cause constipation or upset stomach, but consuming more fiber and drinking more water usually takes care of constipation. If bleeding is quite severe, iron supplements may not be enough, and blood transfusion to replace the lost red cells may be necessary.

Taking iron for anemia and treating bleeding with drugs such as birth control pills often works well enough to eliminate the need for more invasive treatments. First-line treatments for abnormal bleeding include hormones such as progestins or combined oral contraceptives. Bleeding can also be reduced with drugs such as ibuprofen, which are usually given to treat pain. These and other drug treatments are discussed in more detail in chapter 10. In the United Kingdom, progesterone-releasing intrauterine devices, or IUDs, are frequently used to control bleeding, but they are less popular in the United States. Gonadotropin-releasing hormone analogues (GnRH) are much stronger drugs that are sometimes used for short-term treatment of bleeding. Bleeding may sometimes be controlled by uterine fibroid embolization or by a procedure called endometrial ablation, discussed in chapters 11 and 14. As a last resort, bleeding because of fibroids may be controlled by surgery (see chapters 12 and 13).

It's important to understand that fibroids are not the only potential cause of bleeding. In addition to anovulation, endometrial cancer, polyps, and adenomyosis (discussed in the previous chapter), other causes of abnormal bleeding include conditions affecting the ability of blood to clot, such as advanced liver disease or von Willebrand's disease. Undergoing appropriate diagnostic tests should help to identify whether fibroids are the cause of any abnormal bleeding you may be experiencing.

PAIN

Fibroids can be so painful that it becomes difficult to work, have sex, or lead a normal life. About one in three women with fibroids has at least some pelvic pain. Pain from fibroids can occur during periods, or without regard to the menstrual cycle.

Fibroids can cause pain in a number of ways. Probably the most common way is by projecting into the cavity of the uterus, as is typical of the submucosal type of fibroid. The uterus treats submucosal fibroids like a foreign body, the same way an oyster is irritated by a grain of sand within it. The uterus then squeezes as if it's trying to expel this fibroid through the cervix. These uterine muscular contractions are felt as severe cramps, usually during periods. If the fibroids get big enough, they can push against adjacent organs, usually the bladder or rectum. This can be painful as well.

Fibroids can sometimes die or degenerate, causing severe pain. This usually happens with larger fibroids since they are unable to bring in enough blood to keep themselves alive. Imagine the blood supply to a fibroid coming in from the outside of this large ball. The center of the ball is far enough away from these blood vessels that it sometimes doesn't have enough blood to stay alive. The central core of the fibroid then begins to die and, in the process, releases a number of chemicals that spread throughout the bloodstream. These chemicals cause irritation in the uterus and often produce severe pain. As the chemicals spread to other parts of the body, they can cause fever and sometimes flulike symptoms. This process of change in a fibroid is called *red degeneration* or *cell death* and sometimes results in the fibroids being slightly smaller than when they started, but can be very painful. Sometimes medicines containing narcotics, such as morphine, are needed to control this kind of pain.

Red Degeneration/Cell Death

Large fibroids are sometimes unable to get enough blood from the uterus to stay alive. When this happens, the following chain of events occurs:

Lack of adequate blood supply to fibroid

Center of fibroid begins to die

Chemicals created from the death of the fibroid cause irritation and pain in the uterus

Chemicals created from the death of the fibroid spread throughout the bloodstream

Chemicals continue to spread to other parts of the body, causing fever and flulike symptoms

Eventually the pain and symptoms subside, but they sometimes require medical therapies, such as pain relievers or narcotics, to control.

Source: National Uterine Fibroids Foundation.

Pedunculated fibroids can twist on their stalks and degenerate or die from this process. This often results in the sudden onset of severe pain. In some cases, surgery may be needed to remove the fibroid. To control this type of pain, strong prescription drugs are sometimes needed.

Controlling Pain

Many people try to "save pain medication for when they really need it" and take the medicine only when they are in severe pain. This is the worst possible strategy. Pain is much more easily controlled if the medications are taken early in the pain cycle. This means that at the first sign of pain, you should take the maximum dose of pain medication that your doctor recommends. The next doses should be taken based on time (for example, Tylenol is usually taken every four hours) and not on whether the pain returns. Taking pain medication in this way is much more effective than taking it only with severe pain. When pain is severe, even strong pain medications may not control it, but when you take the medicine early, the severe pain can be prevented and you can achieve much better control.

A fear of addiction sometimes keeps people from taking enough pain medication. The rate of addiction to narcotics among people who take them for pain is small. Addicts usually do not become addicted because of the quantity of medication they use, but rather because of a difference in their brain chemistry. The bottom line is, take your medication, take it early, and take it often.

Of course, there are many other causes of pelvic pain besides uterine fibroids. If pain is your primary symptom, it is important that your doctor do a thorough diagnostic evaluation. You don't want to continue taking pain medications for something that is not responding, or for a problem requiring a different approach.

PRESSURE

Abdominal pressure caused by an enlarged uterus can make you very uncomfortable, and it can affect the way your entire body works. To some women, the pressure created by large fibroids feels something like being pregnant. The pressure from large fibroids can also cause incontinence or constipation. If fibroids push against the bladder, they can reduce the amount of urine it can hold, making you have to urinate frequently. Sometimes fibroids cause a condition called *stress incontinence,* in which a small amount of urine leaks every time you laugh, cough, or sneeze.

Fibroids are not the only possible cause of stress incontinence, but they can contribute to it. Kegel exercises, biofeedback, and bladder-training exercises can sometimes help incontinence. Few noninvasive treatments work for the feeling of frequently needing to urinate since it is caused by the physical pressure of fibroids on the bladder. Sometimes gradual training, such as trying to wait a few minutes longer each time before emptying the bladder, works, but you have to be diligent about the training.

In extreme cases, fibroids can compress the tubes called *ureters* that connect the bladder with the kidneys. Fibroids can push the ureters against the bones in the pelvis and slow the normal flow of urine, ultimately causing kidney damage. This is a serious development and absolutely must be treated before both kidneys become compromised. Fortunately, this is a very rare consequence of fibroids, and one that usually happens only if the fibroids are very large. An *intravenous pyelogram* (IVP) can test to see if the ureters are affected by fibroids.

Fibroids growing toward the rectum can press against it and cause constipation by narrowing the space the stool must pass through to get out. Fibroids pressing on the rectum can also cause pain or pressure in the lower back, although low back pain is so common that it's hard to know if fibroids are responsible in most cases. If fibroids push into the vagina, they can make intercourse painful. In the most extreme cases, fibroids can become big enough to make breathing difficult.

BLOATING/FEELING OF FULLNESS

Fibroids can eventually grow quite large, producing a sense of bloating or feeling of fullness and "bulk" visible from the outside, enough to show up in a bathing suit or even normal clothing. A change in body image can be quite distressing even if no other symptoms are present.

The bloating or fullness created by fibroids is not harmful in itself, and it is not necessarily a reason to get treatment. However, some women cannot tolerate this symptom because it makes them feel uncomfortable or because of its impact on the way they look. Treatments that reduce the bulkiness of fibroids include the short-term use of certain drugs, uterine fibroid embolization, and surgery.

SEXUAL DYSFUNCTION

Dyspareunia, pain during sex, is one of the most common complaints heard by gynecologists. Some experts estimate that two-thirds of American women experience dyspareunia at some point during their lives. Dyspareunia can occur before, during, or after intercourse, and repeated instances lead to distress, anxiety, problems within a relationship, and sometimes to sexual avoidance. Dyspareunia can be caused by fibroids, depending on where they are located, but it can be worsened by relationship and/or psychological issues. Individual or couples counseling is often a helpful adjunct to medical treatment.

Fibroids can sometimes get in the way of a normal sex life, and this can be a very distressing symptom. Fibroids are not located in the vagina, except for the rare cervical fibroids, but they can put pressure on the vagina indirectly by pushing against the bladder or rectum. This pressure can make sex uncomfortable, painful, or impossible.

Excessive bleeding, a much more common effect of fibroids, can interfere with sex as well. Fatigue caused by blood loss affects libido, and constant bleeding can certainly reduce your interest in sex. Urinary problems or problems with bowel function, caused by fibroids, can interfere with sexual enjoyment. Libido-depleting depression and anxiety can accompany worries about health problems.

A well-nourished, well-exercised body is more likely to respond to sexual stimulation. Good sex can reduce stress, make your body feel better, and create greater self-esteem. Unfortunately, according to a survey published in the *Journal of the American Medical Association*, more than a third of all American women experience sexual dysfunction at some time in their lives.

Despite how common sexual problems are, doctors don't ask their patients about it nearly enough. One study found that less than half of primary care physicians ask their patients about sexual practices or concerns. This may be because most doctors have less than ten hours of training in medical school on the subject of human sexuality. If you have sexual issues you need to discuss with your doctor, be prepared to bring up the subject. Be as open and honest as possible. Some doctors are quite sympathetic to these issues.

Good medical treatment for fibroids may help control the symptoms responsible for sexual dysfunction, and may improve your sex life. Lifestyle changes will probably give you overall health a boost and make you stronger and more relaxed but sometimes improving sexual problems related to fibroid requires invasive treatment. Fortunately, the vast majority o women who have sexual problems before treatment find that their sex lives improve afterward.

Sex and Uterine Fibroids

There is far too little understood about female sexual function even for women without health problems such as uterine fibroids. Modern investigation into female sexual response began with Masters and Johnson in 1966. They described the four phases of female sexual response, including excitement, plateau, orgasm, and resolution.

For years, there has been debate in the literature about the extent to which female orgasms are related to nerve impulses originating from the clitoris, vagina, and/or uterus. There is evidence that sexual response differs among different women with some experiencing orgasm through one or more nerve pathways.

These differences are significant because of the way different treatments affect the female reproductive tract. For example, nerves leading from the vagina to the cervix are cut during total hysterectomy. As a result, some doctors believe that supracervical hysterectomy (removing only the upper portion of the uterus and leaving the cervix) is less likely to harm normal sexual function, although a recent study showed no difference between women who had supracervical and total hysterectomies. Most other techniques for treating uterine fibroids do not involve removing or cutting major nerve pathways, and so could be expected to have a less dramatic effect on sexual response. Some women, however, have reported sexual dysfunction after uterine fibroid embolization (stopping the blood flow to the fibroids) and after myomectomy (removing only the fibroids).

Because there is so little research on the topic, it is difficult to make definitive statements about the effect of fibroid treatments on sex. Studies of women who have hysterectomy to treat significant gynecologic problems have shown that the majority have improved sex lives after surgery. We have observed the same pattern in our practice. Many women with problems related to fibroids (bleeding, pain, or pelvic fullness or swelling) often have lost interest in sex because they never feel completely well. Whether their problems are relieved by medical treatment or surgery, their sex lives may return to normal.

Some women, however, have new sexual problems after surgery for fibroids. Total hysterectomy with removal of the ovaries is the procedure most commonly associated with these problems. This isn't surprising since removing ovaries in a premenopausal woman produces instant surgical menopause, and lowered ovarian hormone levels can clearly make sex less enjoyable. Lack of estrogen thins the vaginal skin, potentially making sex painful. Loss of ovarian hormones, including estrogen and testosterone, can lower sex drive, and surgical problems can cause pelvic pain.

In general, the better your sex life is before beginning treatment for fibroids, the better it is likely to be after treatment. Women with problems related to sex before surgery may find that their problems remain or worsen after surgery. In most cases, women who are considering invasive treatment for fibroids have significant problems relating to the fibroids. Relieving these problems is likely to improve their sex lives. Avoiding total hysterectomy with ovarian removal would seem to be a sensible step to reduce the likelihood of sexual problems after treatment for fibroids. Myomectomy and uterine fibroid embolization would not generally be expected to cause a decrease in sexual enjoyment, but the likelihood of such problems after such treatment is simply unknown.

INFERTILITY

Couples are usually said to have fertility problems if they have unprotected sex for more than a year without getting pregnant. Perhaps as many as one in every five couples has trouble conceiving a child. Most of the time, fibroids don't affect fertility, and most women with fibroids can get pregnant and carry to term without difficulty. However, fibroids do sometimes cause infertility and can cause problems during pregnancy as well. Needless to say, infertility can be an extraordinarily difficult thing to endure.

Since many women now wish to have children later in life and since fibroids usually occur in the thirties and forties more and more women are dealing with fibroids and pregnancy together. For some women, the problem is getting pregnant; for others, it may be pregnancy-related problems that result from fibroids.

For normal pregnancy to occur, a whole series of interrelated events has to work perfectly. First, sperm are ejaculated into the vagina. From there, they swim through the cervix into the uterine cavity. A combination of the sperm's swimming action and the uterine muscular contractions helps to draw the sperm into the uterus and up into the fallopian tubes. At around the same time, an egg needs to be released from one of the ovaries. The fallopian tube draws the egg inward, pulling it into the cavity of the uterus. Somewhere in the fallopian tube the egg and sperm meet. If the egg is successfully fertilized, the fertilized egg then travels back toward the cavity of the uterus where it implants in the uterine lining. After implanting, this fertilized embryo draws nourishment from the placenta that develops at the site of implantation.

Fibroids can get in the way of this process at a variety of stages. First, fibroids blocking the entrance to the uterus can conceivably block sperm from entering. This is a fairly rare occurrence because fibroids don't usually occur at the cervix, or opening to the uterus. If the sperm make it successfully into the uterus, they have to travel through the cavity of the uterus and into the fallopian tube. Fibroids can occur at the juncture of the tube and the uterus, called the cornual region. These fibroids can block egg fertilization or the passage of a fertilized egg out of the tube and back into the cavity of the uterus. Because nature has created the redundant system of two fallopian tubes, if one is blocked, the other may still function. In some women with multiple fibroids, both tubes may be blocked. Treating this problem usually requires surgery because the physical blockage must be removed.

Submucosal fibroids can also prevent pregnancy by causing inflammation inside the uterus. In this case, a fertilized egg might make its way to the proper location, but the inflammation produced by the fibroids prevents the egg from implanting normally. An IUD prevents pregnancy in a similar way. Fortunately, submucosal fibroids can usually be removed with hysteroscopy, which is one of the less invasive procedures used to treat fibroids.

If the egg and sperm successfully unite and successfully implant in the wall of the uterus, fibroids can still cause problems. If the implantation of this fertilized egg occurs over a fibroid, the blood supply to the growing embryo might be inadequate. When an embryo implants over a fibroid in this manner, the rate of early miscarriage is higher than if it implants over a normal part of the uterus. For most women, this problem won't occur repetitively since the egg implants in a random way over the uterine lining, and the entire lining is probably not littered with fibroids. But for some women, repeated miscarriages early in pregnancy may be the result of fibroids. Again, this problem is best treated by myomectomy in order to remove as many fibroids as possible and leave the uterus in as normal a condition as possible.

Before surgically removing fibroids, all other causes of infertility or miscarriage should be evaluated with a series of tests and studies. For infertility, these tests should include a semen analysis (since half of fertility problems are related to "male factors"), a test to ensure that ovulation is occurring, and a test to see if the fallopian tubes are blocked. Men sometimes resist having their semen tested, but no woman should have major surgery before her partner has had this simple test. Some experienced gynecologists believe that only fibroids within the uterine cavity (submucosal fibroids) associated with two or more miscarriages should be considered for removal. When fibroids are affecting fertility, surgically removing fibroids can greatly increase the chances of pregnancy, although it does not guarantee that pregnancy will occur.

A variety of studies on fertility and myomectomy have been published over the last twenty years. Many of these studies were not well done, meaning that they studied only women who had had myomectomies. This can be a problem because many women with fibroids, if watched long enough, will spontaneously become pregnant. If you study a group of women who have fibroids and are treated with a particular method, you will find that some of them get pregnant, but some proportion of these women would have gotten pregnant even without treatment. Because of this, randomized trials are usually used to try to determine whether a treatment is useful. In a randomized trial, some women are given the treatment and others are given a different treatment or simply watched. By examining how many women in each group become pregnant, observers are better able to tell whether the treatment, or time alone, allowed these women to conceive.

Regardless of the quality of myomectomy studies completed to date, evidence does seem to suggest that having a myomectomy will improve fertility, particularly in women who have no other fertility problems. This means that, after a thorough workup, they have not been found to have other reasons for infertility. A number of studies suggested that about half of women who have fibroids and infertility will be able to get pregnant after a myomectomy. Unfortunately, this does not mean that half will be able to have babies. The rate of spontaneous abortion, as we have seen, is higher in women who have fibroids. Overall, about one-quarter of women who get pregnant after myomectomy actually carry a baby to term. This might sound like a depressing statistic, but it may be higher than the group who had no myomectomy.

It is important when talking to your doctor about these outcomes that you think carefully about the likelihood of pregnancy after treatment. Your doctor might have a skewed view of what constitutes a successful myomectomy. Many physicians reading the literature on this subject conclude that over half of women who have myomectomies have children. Unfortunately, in many cases, they are accepting the pregnancy rate as adequately reflecting the delivery rate. As we have noted, many women who are able to get pregnant are not able to carry children to term. Furthermore, a doctor reflecting on his or her own practice might feel that myomectomy is much more successful than statistics indicate. While a doctor's experience is certainly important, published studies are usually better at providing accurate statistics.

Imagine that we see one hundred women who need myomectomies because they are having trouble getting pregnant, and we believe their fibroids are interfering. Of these hundred, twenty of them might be counseled that, even with a myomectomy, their chances of getting pregnant are very low; possibly because they are over forty or because there is some male-factor infertility involved. This leaves eighty patients. If all of the remaining eighty have myomectomies, we might see only fifty of them for follow-up past their usual six-week postoperative visit. This might be because they have doctors in other areas they normally see or because they didn't like the way we treated them (we certainly hope this number is very low!). Now we're left with fifty patients, of whom let's say about ten decide after their myomectomy that they no longer want to try to have children. Surprisingly, this does happen, even after someone has undergone major surgery. Now let's imagine that twenty patients are able to get pregnant. Our impression might be that half of the patients with myomectomy are able to get pregnant; that's twenty out of forty. But if we look back carefully, we see that only twenty out of eighty have been able to get pregnant, and our experience has been very misleading. This example might sound extreme, but it is exactly the reason published reports of medical treatment place much emphasis on being sure that all the patients who entered the treatment trial are carefully tracked. In our example, that would mean that before we could tell you that half of these patients became pregnant after myomectomy, we would need to go back and investigate what happened to the thirty that never returned to our office. That said, it still seems reasonable to suggest a myomectomy to a woman with infertility and fibroids.

Example Clinical Study of Pregnancy after Myomectomy

Starting point	100 women needing myomectomies because they are having trouble getting pregnant and possibly have interfering fibroids seek surgical assistance and enroll in clinical trial	100 (each figure represents 10 women) 👤👤👤👤👤👤👤👤👤👤
	⬇	
Leave study	20 are told their chances of getting pregnant are very low; possibly because they are over 40 or because some male-factor infertility is involved	Minus 20 👤👤
	⬇	
Surgery	80 patients desiring pregnancy undergo myomectomy	👤👤👤👤👤👤👤👤
	⬇	
Leave study	30 return to referring physician after surgery or seek new care provider	Subtract 30 👤👤👤
	⬇	
	50 patients remain	👤👤👤👤👤
	⬇	
Leave study	10 patients choose not to become pregnant	Subtract 10 👤
	⬇	
	40 patients desiring pregnancy remain	👤👤👤👤
	⬇	
No success	20 patients do *not* become pregnant	Subtract 20 👤👤
	⬇	
Success!	20 patients *do* become pregnant	👤👤

There are some ways to predict who will have a good outcome after myomectomy. A woman's age is a key factor in whether she will be able to get pregnant after myomectomy. In one study of pregnancy after myomectomy, women younger than thirty-five had a conception rate of 62 percent, while older women had a conception rate of only 33 percent. In still another study, not a single woman over the age of thirty-five who had had a myomectomy got pregnant after eighteen months, while 83 percent of women under thirty-five became pregnant within eighteen months.

The number and size of fibroids removed doesn't seem to affect pregnancy rates in women under thirty. In women over thirty, one study showed that women with smaller and less numerous fibroids got pregnant more often. In this study, women who conceived had an average of three fibroids, while those who did not conceive had an average of six fibroids.

Fibroids can grow back after myomectomy, but this usually takes years. Even if the fibroids return, the lag time of several years is usually enough to allow for conception.

Myolysis or cryomyolysis, procedures that cause fibroids to die but don't involve suturing the uterus, are not currently recommended for women wishing to become pregnant since there have been reports of ruptured uteri during pregnancy after these procedures. Uterine fibroid embolization, another new procedure to shrink fibroids, has some promise in this area, particularly for younger women, but it is not currently recommended as a first line of treatment for women who wish to have children. Additional details regarding fertility and embolization are found in chapter 11.

As an alternative treatment, doctors sometimes use drugs called GnRH agonists, such as Lupron, to shrink fibroids temporarily. These drugs are used for about three months, throwing women into a "chemically induced menopause," and causing fibroids to shrink temporarily. Women who use these drugs try to get pregnant in the three to six months following treatment and before the fibroids grow back to their original size after stopping the drugs. This and other medical treatments are covered in detail in chapter 10.

PREGNANCY COMPLICATIONS

About 30 percent of the time, fibroids present at the start of pregnancy may grow larger as pregnancy progresses. However, they cause complications with pregnancy only 10 percent of the time. Complications may include pain, preterm labor, and the need for cesarean delivery.

Fibroids may grow during pregnancy because the body produces much more estrogen and progesterone. It is not known why some fibroids grow during pregnancy while others do not. All fibroids have receptors for estrogen and progesterone, and it may be that those with more receptors will grow most during pregnancy. Most of the time, fibroids that grow don't cause significant problems during pregnancy, and they usually shrink after delivery. There is no way to predict what will happen to a particular fibroid during pregnancy.

Pain

In a study conducted at the University of North Carolina in Chapel Hill, researchers found that only about one in ten pregnant women with fibroids experienced complications during pregnancy. The most common complication was pain, which was easily managed with ibuprofen (Motrin).

Pain during pregnancy sometimes occurs as fibroids suddenly shrink or begin to break down, a process called *degeneration*. Degeneration is the death of muscle cells inside the fibroids. Fibroids may degenerate because as the uterus grows during pregnancy, some of the fibroid's blood supply can be cut off. The pain of a degenerating fibroid is often felt directly over the fibroid. As a fibroid dies, it may also cause pain. Fibroid degeneration typically occurs during the first or second trimester and is sometimes accompanied by fever, nausea, and vomiting. Pain may also be felt over the whole uterus. Since pain during pregnancy may be a sign of premature labor, you should bring any new pain to your obstetrician's attention immediately.

Ultrasound at the site of pain can sometimes determine if a fibroid is the cause. Pain medications and bed rest are typically prescribed as first-line treatments. Symptoms usually go away within a few days. About one-quarter of women with these symptoms have several recurrences later in pregnancy, and these are treated in the same way. If over-the-counter or prescription pain medications don't relieve the pain, women are sometimes hospitalized to receive stronger pain medicine, such as morphine. Surgery during pregnancy is an absolute last resort since it can cause premature labor or result in severe blood loss. Staying in the hospital and receiving pain medication is no picnic. However, for those few women who have severe pain from fibroids in pregnancy, it's probably the best option.

Preterm Labor

Women with uterine fibroids are at higher risk for preterm labor during pregnancy, but almost 90 percent will still deliver at term. In one recent study, the rate of birth at less than thirty eight weeks was almost 8 percent for women without fibroids, but almost 12 percent for women with fibroids. Other studies have shown higher rates of preterm delivery in women with fibroids, with some as high as 20 percent. Babies born to women with fibroids are no more likely to die than are babies born to women without fibroids. They are also no more likely to have significant birth defects than babies born to women without fibroids are. Women who have had previous preterm delivery, who have twins, or who have certain other pregnancy complications are at higher risk of having preterm delivery, and fibroids will probably increase this risk. Very little can be done to prevent preterm delivery in a woman with fibroids.

If you are having preterm labor, your doctor will probably want to keep you in the hospital. Certain medications can be used to slow the onset of labor, although they can't prevent it entirely. Usually the slowing of labor allows enough time to prepare for the birth. In some cases, you can also be given medications that will help speed the baby's lung maturity and reduce the risk of preterm birth complications. Don't let this discussion of preterm birth scare you; as we mentioned, the rate of preterm birth is low, and even if you do have preterm birth, the complication rate is relatively low with modern medical care.

It might seem like having a myomectomy even before you try to get pregnant is always a good idea, but it isn't. A myomectomy carries its own risks, including infertility, so sometimes you might be just as likely to impair your chances of getting pregnant as you would be to improve them.

Cesarean Delivery

Studies have found that women with fibroids are up to six times more likely to need cesarean delivery than are those without fibroids. In a study conducted at the University of North Carolina in Chapel Hill, women with fibroids had a 34 percent rate of cesarean delivery, slightly higher than the hospital's usual rate of 22 percent cesarean births. For the vast majority of women, fibroids sit quietly during pregnancy, but complications can occur.

One reason for the need of cesarean section in women with fibroids has to do with the possibility of fibroids altering the baby's normal position in the uterus. Normally, when labor begins, the baby is positioned with its head pushing against the cervix and its bottom up toward the top of the uterus. If fibroids distort the normal shape of the uterus, this position can be altered and the baby can present in the breech (bottom down) position, or in a sort of sideways orientation. In either case, cesarean delivery will often be necessary.

Fibroids in the lower part of the uterus can also interfere with delivery by preventing normal descent of the fetus through the birth canal. The baby has to squeeze through the maternal pelvis and through the vagina in a space that is not much larger than the baby. You can imagine that jamming a fibroid into this small space would reduce the chance that the baby will fit.

Thankfully, these days cesarean delivery is really not much more complicated than a vaginal delivery. While most people would prefer a vaginal birth, cesarean produces only slightly higher blood loss and slightly longer recovery. In fact, many of us think that cesarean delivery has gotten too good! One reason the cesarean section rate seems to keep increasing year after year is that women and doctors have discovered that the end result of a happy mom and happy baby seems just as likely with cesarean as with vaginal delivery.

If you do require a Cesarean delivery, it might seem like a

good idea to have your fibroids removed at the same time. There is a fair amount of debate about whether this truly is a good idea, and most of it hinges on whether the risks outweigh the benefits. At the time of delivery, the amount of blood flowing to the uterus at any given minute is nearly ten times what it is in the nonpregnant state. This means that a cut made into the uterus will bleed much more quickly at the time of a cesarean than it would at the time of another surgery. Since one of the main complications of myomectomy is excessive blood loss, there is good reason to worry about doing myomectomy at the time of cesarean delivery. On the other hand, you've already had some of the risks of surgery (in other words, you already have your belly cut open), so some of the risks are reduced. It probably is a matter of carefully selecting the right patient for this operation and knowing to quit when you're ahead, should problems arise during the surgery. If several large myomas can be removed at the time of cesarean without much extra bleeding, then it certainly seems worthwhile to do so. For a woman who has many, many myomas, the additional risk of removing them might not be worth taking. In addition, myomas that seem significant at the time of delivery may later shrink. We've seen women with large myomas at the time of cesarean and then gone back and looked with ultrasound many months later and found that those myomas had decreased in size to being almost unnoticeable anymore.

Myomectomy before delivery is almost uniformly a bad idea. The risks to the mother and baby are substantial. Excessive bleeding could seriously harm the baby, and the surgery could initiate preterm labor. However, in rare instances a fibroid degenerating during pregnancy requires treatment. Under this circumstance, surgery may be considered. If you're in this situation, the best you can do is try to find a surgeon who has had experience with this type of operation and have the surgery in a hospital experienced in managing preterm births.

URINARY PROBLEMS

Women with fibroids suffer from urinary problems more frequently than other women do. Fibroids that grow in the front part of the uterus have a tendency to push against the bladder. Even if the fibroids are located in other parts of the uterus, if the combined mass of the fibroids and uterus is big enough, then there could be additional pressure on the bladder. If fibroids or an enlarged uterus push against it, the bladder might be compressed so much that it can only hold 100 cc, or less than half a cup rather than four or five times that amount.

In addition to increasing the frequency of urination, pressure from fibroids can sometimes cause involuntary leakage of urine. Involuntary urine loss affects more than ten million Americans, but many women with incontinence do not talk to their doctor about it, either because they are too embarrassed or because they do not believe that any help is available. Women with incontinence from fibroids usually first notice they leak a small amount of urine when they cough, laugh, or sneeze. As the problem worsens, leaking occurs more and more frequently.

Because both fibroids and bladder problems are common, it's important to make sure the two are actually related before assuming that treating the fibroids will improve the bladder problems. This means that the doctor must take a careful history and do a thorough exam to figure out whether the fibroids are likely to be contributing to the problem. If a history and physical exam are not enough, your doctor may want to order more complicated testing. For any woman who is losing urine involuntarily, the minimum test that should be done is a urine culture to make sure no infection is present. Your doctor may also want to order something called urodynamics. As part of this test, the bladder is filled with water and the amount of water held before feeling the urge to go is measured. Also, any leaking of urine can be observed directly.

We have found that bladder problems that were evaluated before surgery and found to be likely related to fibroids resolve about 70 percent of the time after myomectomy or hysterectomy. Unfortunately, there is no similar data about the resolution of these kinds of problems after uterine fibroid embolization or other treatments.

DEPRESSION

While physical symptoms may be the most common reason women with fibroids seek treatment, psychological problems such as depression and anxiety may also lead women to seek a doctor's help. Health problems increase emotional stress and feelings of loneliness and isolation. Stress may come from having to handle an additional problem in an already overburdened life or from tension over how to handle fibroids. Many women who decide against hysterectomy find their mothers or friends unable to understand their choice, and this can be an isolating feeling. If fibroids are causing you a lot of mental anguish, you may want to consult a counselor or psychologist who is trained to help people resolve emotional issues. Your gynecologist may not be the best person to handle these issues, but local mental health centers often offer counseling on a sliding scale, and many churches and synagogues have trained lay counselors who can talk to you. Support groups can be found through local health resources and on the Internet. It is very important to discuss your feelings with your doctor. Even if he or she can't help you with your emotional issues, your doctor should at least listen patiently. If he or she does not appreciate your situation or ignores your complaints, you should find another doctor.

When your doctor and you have evaluated your symptoms, the next decision is whether to treat your fibroids, and if so, which treatment to use. The choice of treatment should be made in partnership with your doctor, but the decision is ultimately yours. The most conservative strategy, watchful waiting, a first step for many women in this process, is covered in the next chapter.

Chapter 5

Watchful Waiting

Since fibroids are benign tumors, you usually have time to monitor their progress for a while before choosing a treatment. Although fibroids grow over time, they can also stabilize or shrink, particularly after menopause. A period of what is called "watchful waiting" gives you a chance to assess how bad your fibroids make you feel, think about your treatment options, and ultimately choose the option that is best for you.

Returning to your doctor's office to check the size of your fibroids is a sensible first step. Watchful waiting is *unquestionably* the best strategy if you have no symptoms from fibroids, or if symptoms are not particularly troublesome. However, if your symptoms are unbearable, you will want to treat them right away. Watchful waiting is of no use if you are already suffering and know you cannot continue without some improvement in your symptoms. If this describes you, you can safely skip this chapter and move right to the chapters dealing with treatment.

TREATING FIBROIDS

Primum no nocere means "First, do no harm." The distinguished Greek physician Hippocrates put forth this most important principle of medicine more than a thousand years ago, and it is relevant to the treatment of fibroids. One of our professors once observed, "It's hard to make someone feel better if they feel fine to begin with." Or, more simply stated, "If it ain't broke, don't fix it." If you have no symptoms from fibroids, or if you can live just fine with them, then don't let anybody scare you into having your uterus, or anything else, removed.

Suddenly finding out that you have fibroids inside your body may have frightened you. Your fear may be pushing you to "do something," and to do it now. After all, this is an action-oriented society. Although your doctor may counsel patience, you may be the kind of person who is already obsessively thinking about how to get rid of those fibroids. You may want to get rid of them immediately, even before you understand your treatment options. This anxiety and stress can be overwhelming.

One way to keep things in perspective after you've just been diagnosed with fibroids is to ask yourself, "Before I knew I had fibroids, did I have a problem?" If the answer is no, you don't need invasive treatment yet. In fact, you may not need any treatment at all. With the high-quality ultrasound and MRI scans available, many women without symptoms discover they have fibroids simply because they've had one of these tests. Watchful waiting is the only sensible plan if this describes your situation.

EVALUATING SYMPTOMS

All treatment decisions must ultimately be made by you, in consultation with your doctor. It is your doctor's responsibility to explain your options, but it is your responsibility to understand them and to make choices regarding your own health. How you choose to proceed with medical treatment is a highly personal decision. It is very important for you to think carefully about all of your options and consider how your symptoms affect your life.

Common sense demands that you try the least invasive treatments first. If your symptoms are tolerable, conservative treatment strategies such as lifestyle modifications or medications should be your first steps. Modifying your diet, beginning an exercise program, and beginning a stress reduction program are low-risk interventions that will improve your overall health and may help control your symptoms, even if they don't shrink your fibroids. Drug treatments are effective on many women. Birth control pills and painkillers such as Tylenol or ibuprofen are low-risk treatments. Alternative medicine, covered in chapter 9, helps some women control symptoms.

If less risky interventions have been given a fair trial and failed, a new therapy called *uterine fibroid embolization* (UFE) is one of the least invasive of the major interventions. Surgeries such as *myomectomy*, which removes fibroids but retains the uterus, and *hysterectomy*, which removes both the fibroids and the uterus, are more invasive than UFE, but may be better choices for some women. Invasive procedures offer the best chance of controlling symptoms but also carry the highest risk of complications.

You must base your decision on how to treat fibroids on

your own individual symptoms. For instance, if you notice that your pants are not fitting as well, or if you have some bloating because of fibroids, think about exactly how bothersome these symptoms are to you. Are your symptoms easily ignored, completely unbearable, or somewhere in between?

We have seen many women who cannot leave their homes for four or five days a month due to heavy menstrual bleeding. Some of these women also have severe pain for a day or two a month, but otherwise they function beautifully. How should these women treat their fibroids? Does this inconvenience and reduced level of functioning justify something as invasive as a hysterectomy? These are important questions. But they are not questions a doctor can answer. The answers depend on each woman's tolerance of her symptoms. If you have cancer, a doctor might tell you, "Without this surgery you have a life expectancy of five years; with it, twenty-five years." For most people, the decision in this case is an easy one. With fibroids, the choices are usually much more subtle. Except in rare cases, treating fibroids won't add one day to your life—but it may make the days you have much more enjoyable. Rarely, treating fibroids *is* about lengthening your life. For example, if you have severe anemia despite treatment, you must seriously consider invasive treatments. Anemia can truly shorten your life. Not only might anemia cause you to lose consciousness and have an accident, but your risk of heart attack and stroke rises if your blood count falls too low. These outcomes are rare enough that the vast majority of women with fibroids have the luxury, along with the burden, of choosing whether to live with their symptoms or when to undertake invasive treatment.

MANAGING SYMPTOMS

The three levels of treatment for fibroids are listed here beginning with the most conservative:

1. *Lifestyle changes* include strategies to improve your diet, increase physical exercise, and reduce stress. Lifestyle changes are very safe and can easily be combined with medical treatment, but they are slow to take effect and require some patience. In many women, lifestyle changes may have little or no effect on fibroid growth or fibroid-related symptoms, but these changes have benefits that go beyond improving the symptoms from fibroids, such as lowering your blood pressure or cholesterol. See chapters 6, 7, and 8 for specific suggestions on lifestyle changes.

2. *Medical (as opposed to surgical) treatments* include drug treatments for symptoms, and complementary therapies such as Chinese medicine or acupuncture. These can have a more dramatic effect on symptoms than lifestyle changes, although symptoms often return after therapy is stopped. In addition, use of pharmaceuticals and nutraceuticals are reversible decisions, unlike surgical therapies. Generally, prescription drug treatments have undergone much more rigorous scientific testing of their usefulness than alternative approaches. Chapters 9 and 10 cover medical treatments.

3. *Invasive therapies* include uterine fibroid embolization, myomectomy, and hysterectomy. These have an immediate effect on symptoms, but are usually the riskiest treatments. See chapters 11, 12, and 13 for more information on invasive therapies.

MONITORING FIBROIDS

When your doctor discovers that you have fibroids, one of the first things he or she may do is to note the approximate size of your fibroid uterus. Next, an ultrasound or MRI more accurately defines the size and number of your fibroids. These medical records become a *baseline* against which fibroids may be measured on the next visit. From this starting point, your doctor can determine whether the fibroids are growing, remaining stable in size, or shrinking. Monitoring the growth of fibroids for a few office visits is a prudent approach followed by most doctors. Unless you have significant symptoms, a doctor recommending treatment based on one exam should be a warning flag. Fibroids usually grow slowly. Repeating the exam three to six months after the fibroids are initially diagnosed is a good strategy.

If your fibroids are growing rapidly, they should be monitored more frequently until the growth subsides or you are comfortable in choosing a treatment. Many doctors tell women that rapidly growing fibroids "may be cancer" and should be removed rather than monitored. Those doctors may not know that Dr. William Parker and his colleagues performed a study that pretty much laid to rest this theory. They found that about three out of every thousand women operated on for fibroids had cancer, whether the fibroids were growing quickly or not. The study concluded that uterine cancer was not predictable and confirmed that it is very rare. Treating a problem as common as fibroids with surgery to find the rare uterine cancer is a risky approach, since doing so many operations might injure more women than it saves.

Missing a diagnosis of cancer in the early stages is the greatest single risk of watchful waiting, and every doctor's and patient's worst nightmare. Fortunately, your doctor can rule out the most common types of cancer with a fair amount of certainty. Annual Pap smears can rule out cervical cancer, an endometrial biopsy (described in chapter 3) can rule out endometrial cancer, and ultrasound or MRI along with CA-125 tests can reduce the risk that ovarian cancer may be missed.

In our opinion, simply having big fibroids is not reason enough to undergo treatment. Many doctors have been taught that when the uterus reaches the size of a twelve-week pregnancy, it is time for a hysterectomy. There are no sound, scientifically based reasons to support doing a hysterectomy on a woman who simply has big fibroids and no troublesome symptoms. One rationalization given for this approach is that big fibroids make it difficult for doctors to perform a thorough pelvic exam, and they may miss an ovarian cancer as a result. Ovarian cancer is a serious concern, but transvaginal ultrasound, CT scans, and MRI tests are good ways to check for ovarian cancer. In cases in which the ovaries are found to be normal with ultrasound, the incidence of ovarian cancer is quite low. Ovarian cancer is quite difficult to detect in the early stages even when fibroids are *not* present and even using the most sophisticated tests available. The benefits and risks of surgically removing the ovaries to prevent ovarian cancer are covered in greater detail in chapter 13, but removing fibroids just so your doctor can more easily perform a pelvic exam strikes us as ridiculous. You wouldn't take your front door off its hinges to make it easier to bring in groceries, would you? Why not just check the ovaries another way, such as with ultrasound, and leave the uterus alone?

Another rationalization for removing big fibroids is that the risks of surgery are less when fibroids are smaller. Or as many doctors say "Let's get them out now, before they get any bigger." Although this seems logical, it is just not true. In 1992 a pioneering study by Robert Reiter, M.D., of the University of Iowa College of Medicine demonstrated that surgical complications are no greater for women with larger fibroids than they are for women with smaller fibroids. Another rationalization for recommending hysterectomy to women with no symptoms is to prevent symptoms such as bleeding or pain from ever occurring. Having surgery for a nonexistent problem is a little like giving away your car because you're afraid you might have an accident.

You can continue watchful waiting as long as your symptoms are not bothering you. The younger you are when diagnosed, the longer you may have to wait and the more likely your fibroids are to grow before menopause.

MENOPAUSE

Fibroids often stop growing after menopause, when hormone levels drop. There is no accurate way to predict when a particular woman will enter menopause. In the United States it usually happens sometime between the ages of forty and sixty, and about 50 percent of women enter menopause by age fifty-one.

Menopause means "the last period," and since this cannot be identified until after it occurs and is followed by a year of no periods, the entire time when periods are becoming less regular is often called "the menopausal transition" or even "perimenopause." This transition is a gradual process, and one that involves many hormonal changes in a woman's body. Fundamentally, this represents a change from the time when a woman can have children and when she cannot. Some women experience menopause as "a time of loss," some as a "passage" into greater wisdom and maturity, and some as a combination of the two.

Menopause often brings physical changes and swings in mood. About one-third of women have bothersome symptoms including hot flashes, night sweats, sleeping problems, and vaginal dryness. Psychological symptoms can include a lower interest in sex, depression, and anxiety. Most women don't have significant problems when they become menopausal, and may find the lack of periods and cyclic hormone surges to be a relief. Furthermore, because of declining estrogen levels in the body, fibroids usually shrink after menopause.

Knowing the age when your female relatives entered menopause can give you some basis to guess when you might enter menopause. If your mother and grandmother both entered menopause at the age of fifty, for instance, it's likely that you will begin menopause at about that age too. A blood test for a hormone called follicle-stimulating hormone, or FSH, can also give some idea of whether you are close to menopause. This hormone, produced in the brain, tells your ovaries how much estrogen to make. As the ovaries begin to slow down the production of estrogen (a sign of menopause), the brain makes more and more FSH, as if shouting louder and louder at the ovaries in the hope they will hear. If the FSH level has started to rise, it suggests that menopause is approaching. If you have symptoms from fibroids and menopause seems to be around the corner, you might be able to wait it out and avoid treatment altogether.

Drugs or medications can sometimes shrink fibroids and control symptoms, but may be harmful if used for longer term. (Medical therapies are covered in detail in chapter 10.) The closer you are to menopause, the easier it is to decide whether this brief respite will be enough. Unfortunately, even knowing a family history and checking the FSH level, won't allow a doctor to predict when a particular woman may enter menopause since FSH rises unpredictably. That is, your FSH may be high, suggesting that menopause is *near*, but does *near* mean two months, six months, or two years? No one knows, and although many doctors have tried to work out formulas for predicting when the last period will come, none of them works very well.

WATCHFUL WAITING

Watchful waiting is really just the process of monitoring the fibroids, and it's a good strategy unless you already have symptoms that need treatment. After establishing a baseline, your doctor can tell you if your fibroids are growing, but only you can determine how much your symptoms bother you. If symptoms are mild, try lifestyle changes and conservative medical treatment options before proceeding to more risky and permanent procedures. Menopause may bring relief from fibroids, although it is difficult to predict when menopause will occur.

When Is Watchful Waiting a Good Idea?

- Baseline established using ultrasound or MRI
- Symptoms are tolerable
- No significant anemia
- Fibroids are not causing excessive bleeding
- Other conditions ruled out
  —Pap smear
  —Endometrial biopsy

Chapter 6

Diet

Medical treatments for fibroids work best in the context of a healthy lifestyle. Lifestyle changes covered in the next few chapters involve not only a good diet, the topic of this chapter, but also exercise and stress reduction. These lifestyle changes will not produce immediate results, but will dramatically strengthen body and mind over time.

Controversy exists over the role of diet in treating women with symptomatic fibroids. We discuss many studies in this chapter that suggest possible links among diet, estrogen, and fibroids. However, clear proof of any direct links is still lacking. Changes in diet may help slow the growth of fibroids, but dietary changes are more often useful in helping to moderate symptoms such as bleeding or pain. This chapter recommends a basic healthy diet for women with fibroids, including foods, vitamins, and minerals that may help with specific symptoms.

Following a good, sound, well-balanced diet including protein, whole grains, fruits, and vegetables is undeniably good for your overall physical and mental health. What you eat is important, since food powers every move you make.

Most of the foods recommended in this chapter are not of animal origin. Even so, although some studies have shown that women who eat less red meat are less likely to develop symptomatic fibroids, there are no studies that demonstrate that fibroid growth can be stopped by altering your diet.

> J.C., thirty-four, was suffering from very excessive bleeding triggered by several growing fibroids. She became a vegetarian, having heard that it might help control her bleeding and help her avoid a hysterectomy. Although it took a lot of self-discipline, she says, "When I became a complete vegetarian, I had a lot less bleeding. I went from eight to nine days a month of very heavy bleeding down to six to seven days a month of normal bleeding." While a vegetarian diet did not make the fibroids go away, it helped her keep her bleeding under control for several years.

Women who avoid meat and eat more fish, whole grains, and vegetables tend to live longer and healthier lives. A recent study reported in the *New England Journal of Medicine* demonstrated that people who eat fish once a week have about a third lower death rate from heart problems. Previous studies have shown similar effects. Numerous studies have linked a diet high in whole grains and vegetables to lower blood pressure, lower risk of colon cancer, and even lower risk of breast cancer.

It's not clear, however, whether the diets are truly responsible for these health effects because people with healthy diets tend to be healthy people. In other words, some skeptics argue that people who are healthy to begin with are more likely to adopt a good diet. This makes it appear as though the diet alone reduces the risk of those health problems, when in fact it might not be the case. While proving that changes in diet reduce the risk of all these problems is difficult, the overwhelming body of evidence seems to support this idea. Studies of people moving from areas whose inhabitants enjoy a healthy diet to areas where an unhealthy diet prevails also support this idea. Indeed, studies have shown an increased risk of heart disease and cancer when people move to places with less healthy diets.

In this chapter we do not want to suggest that eating certain foods will make your fibroids go away. Instead, we want to support the idea that a healthy diet will improve the strength of your body to fight off any problems it encounters. Eating well will make you less susceptible to problems related to stress, will improve your long-term health, and may reduce your symptoms. A diet directed at your specific problems might also help reduce pain and counteract the effects of severe bleeding. Remember, changing your diet is not easy. Your best chance may be to make gradual changes, reducing the amount of red meat in your diet, or reducing saturated fats and nutritionally empty calories bit by bit. A gradual change you maintain over time will be better for you than rapid changes you soon abandon.

Some medical doctors are very nutritionally oriented and may provide useful advice. Others are frankly clueless. The medical use of food is called *clinical nutrition*, and there are medical doctors who actually specialize in this. Practitioners of naturopathic medicine may also be well trained in dietary strategies for preventing and controlling disease. Some chiropractors, practitioners of Ayurvedic medicine, and other alternative practitioners focus heavily on diet. Registered dietitians can help you plan balanced, nutritious meals, but do not usually make special diets for women with fibroids. Be careful when choosing a counselor to help you plan a healthy diet. Calling yourself a nutritionist doesn't require any actual training or education in nutrition. Some nutritional practitioners may offer advice that could be considered unsound or even dangerous.

A HEALTHY DIET

A good, healthy diet for women with fibroids is very similar to a diet for people who wish to avoid heart disease and other chronic illness. Dietary suggestions made in this chapter are based on a combination of dietary research done on women with fibroids or bleeding disorders and nutritionally balanced diets generally recommended for a wide variety of chronic illnesses. For most women with fibroids, we suggest the following general dietary guidelines:

- Increase your consumption of plant foods, especially vegetables, and particularly green leafy vegetables rich in iron.
- Lower your consumption of red meat, including beef or ham, and increase your consumption of fish.
- Eat plenty of fiber, particularly whole grains, legumes, fruits, and vegetables.
- Reduce your consumption of processed or highly refined foods containing large amounts of saturated fat, salt, or sugar.
- Reduce your intake of highly sugared drinks.

There are two things, discussed in more detail later in this chapter, we don't think you need to worry about when seeking a diet to help your symptoms:

- Reducing your coffee drinking
- Drinking six to eight glasses of water a day

In late 1999 a large research study in Italy strongly suggested that what you eat might correlate with the *development* of symptomatic fibroids. In this groundbreaking study published in *Obstetrics and Gynecology*, Italian scientists matched the diets of approximately 800 women who had surgery for fibroids against the diets of 1,500 women with no history of fibroids or fibroid surgery. The Italian researchers found that women who consumed the highest levels of beef, ham, and other red meat—and ate fewer vegetables, fruits, and fish—had much higher rates of fibroids.

The researchers concluded that women who ate beef had a 70 percent higher risk of fibroids, when compared with women whose diets contained the least meat. Women who ate the most vegetables had a 50 percent lower risk of fibroids than did women who ate the least vegetables. Milk, liver, carrots, eggs, cheese, whole grain foods, butter, margarine, and oil were not associated with symptomatic fibroids in this study. Coffee, tea, and alcohol use were also not associated with symptomatic fibroids.

The Italian scientists speculated that high levels of estrogen-like chemicals contained in some meats could spur the growth of fibroids. Conversely, they speculated that eating fruits and vegetables might actually lower the estrogen level in blood. A good diet, of course, may also be an indicator of an overall healthy lifestyle. It may be this lifestyle, rather than diet, that led to lower rates of symptomatic fibroids in these women.

Another study, published in the *Journal of the National Cancer Institute* in 1981, found that women who are vegetarians do actually have lower levels of estrogen, as well as higher levels of a substance called *sex hormone binding globulin*, which has the effect of pulling excess hormones from the blood. Researchers speculated that differences in hormone levels between vegetarian and nonvegetarian women might explain lower rates of endometrial and breast cancer in vegetarian women. Like fibroids, endometrial and breast cancer are estrogen dependent, so this study gives a possible explanation for the link between vegetarianism and low rates of symptomatic fibroids.

The combined research from all of these studies begins to build a believable picture of some relationship between diet and symptomatic fibroids. This is not really surprising, if you consider that diet can affect your risk of heart attack, the level of your blood pressure, and your risk of certain kinds of cancer. None of these studies suggested that becoming a vegetarian will affect fibroids that already exist. However, it might be reasonable to consider that these dietary changes could reduce the growth of existing fibroids and possibly prevent new ones from forming.

ESTROGEN

Women in socioeconomically developed countries are exposed to many estrogen-like or estrogen-modifying chemicals in the diet, which is a relatively new phenomenon in human history. Some doctors believe that these so-called *xenoestrogens* (*xeno* means "foreign") may be linked to high levels of breast cancer, prostate cancer, and other health problems such as fibroids. Many dieticians accept the idea that a diet high in saturated fats and dairy products elevates estrogen levels.

Meat, poultry, and farmed fish may contain high levels o

steroid hormones such as synthetic estrogens. Animals raised for consumption are often given these substances to make them gain weight. Many animals in this country, particularly cows, are fattened by steroid injections. These injections cause the animals to gain weight more quickly. Animals that gain weight quickly are brought to market sooner, which brings down the price of meat. Some authorities believe that high consumption of xenoestrogens may be responsible for many hormone-dependent cancers such as breast cancer, uterine cancer, and prostate cancer, although this cancer link is far from proven.

Before you take drastic steps to attempt to reduce xenoestrogens in your diet, remember that there is little reliable evidence linking them to fibroids, cancer, or anything else. The concerns are based on theories. Theories, even reasonable ones, are not the same as evidence. If you want to do something with your diet proven to improve your health, eliminate highly processed foods, reduce your fat consumption, and eat more fresh fruits and vegetables.

LOW-FAT, HIGH-FIBER DIETS

We recommend a vegetable-rich, low in fat, high in fiber diet for women with fibroids. Unfortunately, people these days are pressured for time, with little time to prepare good meals. Perhaps as a result, the average U.S. diet contains too much processed food, which is chemically different and less nutritious than food in a more natural state.

Eating a high-fiber diet may help with constipation and bloating by clearing the bowel and reducing pressure in the pelvic area. Foods high in fiber are usually nutritious, since processing removes fiber along with vitamins and minerals, and often adds sugar and salt. Some excellent sources of both fiber and nutrients are whole grains, legumes, vegetables, fruits, seeds, and nuts. High-fiber diets may even reduce the body's overall estrogen exposure. An article published in the *New England Journal of Medicine* concluded that whole grains help the body absorb estrogen and carry it away in the bowel.

Whole grains such as oats, brown rice, and buckwheat are excellent sources of fiber, as well as B vitamins and vitamin E. Whole wheat flour has much more fiber than white flour. Legumes, including soybeans and soybean products, are good sources of fiber and are high in iron, so they help combat the anemia caused by blood loss sometimes associated with fibroids.

Vegetables in the diet are a good source of fiber and contain minerals such as calcium, magnesium, and potassium, along with vitamins. Many vegetables such as Brussels sprouts, broccoli, peppers, potatoes, and peas are high in vitamin C. Low vitamin C levels have been linked to poor wound healing and bleeding problems, so it makes sense to get enough in your diet. Diets high in vegetables and low fat calcium-rich foods such as low-fat cottage cheese have been shown to lower blood pressure. The DASH (Dietary Approaches to Stop Hypertension) diet is widely recommended by physicians and medical groups as a sound dietary approach to balancing nutrient intake while controlling weight gain and hypertension. This diet is one of the few scientifically proven to improve your health.

Dash Diet

Food Group	Daily Servings	Serving Sizes	Suggested Examples
Grains	7–8	1 slice bread ½ cup dry cereal ½ cup cooked rice, pasta, or cereal	Bagel Cereal English muffin Grits Oatmeal Pita bread Whole grain wheat
Vegetables	4–5	1 cup raw, leafy vegetable ½ cup cooked vegetable 6 ounces vegetable juice	Artichokes Beans Broccoli Carrots Collards Kale Peas Potatoes Spinach Squash Sweet potatoes Tomatoes Turnip greens
Fruits	4–5	¼ cup dried fruit ½ cup fresh, frozen, or canned fruit 1 medium fruit 6 ounces fruit juice	Apricots Bananas Dates Grapefruit Grapefruit juice Grapes Mangoes Melons Orange juice Oranges Peaches Pineapples Prunes Raisins Strawberries Tangerines

Food Group	Daily Servings	Serving Sizes	Suggested Examples
Dairy, low-fat or nonfat	2–3	1 cup yogurt 1.5 ounces cheese 8 ounces milk	Buttermilk, skim, or low-fat Cheese, nonfat Milk, skim or 1% Mozzarella cheese Yogurt, nonfat or low-fat
Meats, poultry, and fish	2	3 ounces cooked	Lean meat with all visible fat trimmed; broiled, roasted, or boiled All skin from poultry removed
Nuts, seeds, and legumes	4–5 per week	½ cup cooked legumes ½ ounce or 2 tablespoons seeds 1.5 ounces or ⅓ cup nuts	Almonds Filberts Kidney beans Lentils Mixed nuts Peanuts Sunflower seeds Walnuts

Source: U.S. Department of Health and Human Services, National Heart, Lung and Blood Institute, March 2001.

Fruits contain many nutrients including vitamin C and bioflavonoids. These nutrient chemicals, which give fruits their color, may also help normalize estrogen levels. Many fruits including bananas, figs, and raisins are good sources of potassium, calcium, and magnesium. Fresh fruit is nutritionally superior to canned fruit or fruit juice products, which have less fiber and more sugar.

If you do increase your intake of fiber, you should also increase the amount of water you drink since water is necessary to move fiber through the body. Drinking enough water reduces the risk of kidney stones and possibly bladder infections. Strangely, even though many health experts recommend drinking six to eight glasses of water a day, Dr. Heinz Valtin, a noted water researcher, recently pointed out that there is no scientific evidence to support this claim. Rather the "8x8" myth (eight glasses, eight ounces each) probably started from the misreading of a government publication from 1945. This document noted that while most people needed about sixty-four ounces of water a day, the majority of it could be obtained in foods. Ignoring the high water content of many foods, some took this advice to mean that everyone should drink at least sixty-four ounces of water a day. Better research shows that drinking enough so you are not thirsty is more than enough.

Since coffee and tea are diuretics, many people believe they actually remove water from the body. Research has shown, however, that even coffee and tea are adequate for your normal fluid needs. The diuretic effect of these drinks just means you would have to drink eight ounces of coffee to get the same amount of fluid as four to six ounces of water. Sugar-laden juices, juice drinks, and sodas are sources of excessive calories, so if you are trying to lose weight, skip these drinks.

As you add more fiber to your diet, you may find yourself naturally reducing your consumption of foods such as red meat, which are high in saturated fat. Diets high in saturated fat may cause higher levels of estrogen to circulate in the body. An analysis of thirteen different scientific studies published in the *Journal of the National Cancer Institute* in 1999 concluded that women who reduced their intake of fats could also significantly reduce the levels of estrogen in their blood. The greatest reductions in estrogen levels occurred in two studies in which dietary fat was reduced most, to between 10 and 12 percent of total calories. The estradiol form of estrogen was reduced an average of 13 percent in these studies—7.4 percent among women who had not begun menopause and 23 percent among postmenopausal women. While this reduction has not been proven to help fibroids, reducing fat intake is healthful, so these types of diet changes are worth trying.

PHYTOESTROGENS

Some dieticians recommend eating more foods containing *phytoestrogens*. These are weak estrogens derived from plants (*phyto* means "plant"). In theory, phytoestrogens reduce natural estrogen by competing with it in the body. Phytoestrogens are believed to bind to receptors for estrogen, thereby blocking the effects of the body's own stronger estrogens. Unlike fat-soluble xenoestrogens, phytoestrogens are water soluble and easily eliminated from the body.

Phytoestrogens are found in legumes, including various types of beans such as soy, pinto, garbanzo, and black beans. Phytoestrogens are also found in clover and alfalfa. Cruciferous vegetables such as cabbage, broccoli, cauliflower, Brussels sprouts, kale, mustard greens, collard greens, bok choy, and turnips all contain phytoestrogens as well. These vegetables also contain indoles, enzymes in the body that deactivate estrogen. Indoles convert the strongest form of estrogen, estradiol, into the milder form, called estrone. *Isoflavones*, a type of phytoestrogen, are found in soy and many other legumes. In theory, isoflavones counteract excessive estrogen in the body by crowding out more potent forms of estrogens. Isoflavones also promote bone formation and may reduce the risk of heart disease.

Soybeans contain another phytoestrogen called *genistein*, an antioxidant that also helps normalize estrogen levels. Soy based foods may reduce the severity of menopausal symptoms including hot flashes and vaginal dryness. One concern about increasing soy in the diet is that soybeans are among the most heavily bioengineered products in the world. Approximately 80 percent of all soybeans consumed in the United States are genetically modified (GMO), so if the idea of eating bioengineered foods bothers you, try to select GMO-free soy products.

FOODS THAT MAY HELP BLEEDING

Women with heavy bleeding lose significant quantities of iron, which the body cannot make on its own. Without iron, the body cannot replace the lost red blood cells, so eating foods containing iron helps your body respond to the bleeding caused by fibroids.

Foods that increase the level of easily absorbable, or *heme*, iron in the diet include meat, poultry, and fish. Salmon is relatively high in heme iron and is a good choice for women who want to avoid red meat. Because heme iron comes from animal foods, vegetarians need another source of iron. Other foods contain less well absorbed, nonheme iron. These include eggs, dairy products, dark green leafy vegetables, beans, peas, fruits, nuts, and seeds. Brewer's yeast, wheat germ, and blackstrap molasses are also rich natural sources of iron. Eating foods containing vitamin C, such as broccoli, citrus fruits, melons, tomatoes, and strawberries, increases the absorption of nonheme iron. Eating one orange with a meal is said to double the amount of nonheme iron your body can absorb from plant foods.

Iron Supplements

One confusing thing about increasing iron in your diet is that iron in foods is usually measured as "elemental" iron, but iron in supplements is described by the total amount of iron. For example, in a 325-milligram tablet of ferrous sulfate, one of the most common forms of iron supplements, there are only 65 mg of elemental iron. Nonpregnant women without heavy blood loss need only about 18 mg of elemental iron a day in their diets, but women who are bleeding might need as much as 125 mg of elemental iron a day.

Iron Content of Some Common Foods and Supplements

Food/Supplement	Serving Size	Milligrams (mg) Elemental Iron
Broccoli	3.5 oz	1.1 mg
Eggs	1	1.5 mg
Tofu	3.5 oz	1.8 mg
Pistachios	1 oz	1.9 mg
Spinach	3.5 oz	2.7 mg
Hamburger	3.5 oz	2.7 mg
Beans	3.5 oz	3 mg
Liver	3.5 oz	5.7 mg
Ferrous gluconate	325 mg	37 mg
Ferrous sulfate	325 mg	65 mg
Ferrous fumigate	200 mg	66 mg

Vitamins

Vitamin A, an antioxidant, may help control excessive bleeding. In one study, forty women who suffered excessive bleeding took 60,000 IU of vitamin A per day for thirty-five days. More than 90 percent of the women showed some decrease in bleeding. Vitamin A returned almost 60 percent of the women to normal periods for at least three months after supplementation. Another 35 percent of these women saw a reduction in blood loss for the duration of their periods, while 7.5 percent of participants had no effect.

Unfortunately, these studies had no control group—a group of women who took only sugar or placebo pills—so some of the improvement may have been a result of chance alone. In addition, the studies did not look specifically at women with fibroids, just at women with excessive menstrual bleeding. There is no guarantee that the results would be the same in women with fibroids, but reasonable amounts of supplemental vitamin A are safe to try. A recent study found that too much vitamin A increases the risk of osteoporosis, so don't overdo it! Carrots, sweet potatoes, spinach, dried apricots, liver, fish, and dairy products (fortified) are high in vitamin A.

Vitamin C, an important antioxidant that increases iron absorption, has many roles in the body, including an ability to strengthen very small blood vessels called capillaries. Tears in these small vessels may contribute to excessive bleeding. One research study showed that almost 90 percent of women who were given vitamin C achieved reductions in excessive bleeding. Again, this study was not controlled (there was no comparison group), so some of that improvement may have been from chance alone. Taking at least 1 gram or 1,000 mg per day or more, in divided doses, is often recommended for antioxidant purposes. Red peppers, guava, kale, broccoli, Brussels sprouts, cauliflower, persimmons, citrus fruits, and strawberries are among the foods high in vitamin C.

Vitamin K, found in green leafy vegetables, wheat grass, alfalfa, and other green juices containing chlorophyll, helps blood clot. Deficiencies of vitamin K are quite rare; however, some nutritionists recommend supplements of 150–500 micrograms per day for women with bleeding. Turnip greens, broccoli, lettuce, cabbage, beef liver, spinach, and asparagus are high in vitamin K.

Vitamins to Treat Fibroids

Along with alternative treatments, herbs, and other complementary therapies, women have considered trying to use vitamins to treat fibroid-related problems or to prevent fibroids from growing. Unfortunately, there is very little evidence that inadequate vitamin intake has anything to do with fibroid-related problems. There is even less evidence that taking vitamin supplements will reduce the problems.

This doesn't mean that vitamins have no value, however. In some very small groups of women, inadequate vitamin K, for example, may result in problems with bleeding. It is very rare for normal women to have inadequate vitamin K unless they have very unusual diets or significant health problems. Inadequate vitamin B_{12} can also lead to anemia, which can be made worse by bleeding problems related to fibroids, but B_{12} deficiency is rare except in alcoholics.

For most women, vitamins are not a useful treatment for fibroids, but they may be helpful in preventing or treating other conditions, particularly if they are absorbed in the form of food rather than supplements. A recent article in the *Journal of the American Medical Association* reviewed the evidence surrounding vitamin treatment for common conditions (Fairfield, JAMA 2002; 287:3,116–3,126). For women, vitamin D is probably the most important vitamin to pay attention to. Many women have inadequate vitamin D intake, and this has been associated with osteoporosis. Vitamin D needs to be taken in the presence of adequate calcium in order for it to help improve bone density, and women need 1,200–1,500 mg of calcium per day. This much calcium can be obtained from three to five servings of low-fat dairy products or from supplements.

Women of childbearing age should consider taking folic acid (also called folate) supplements. There is a clear relationship between inadequate folate intake during pregnancy and increased risk of neural tube defects in the developing fetus. Specifically, women with low folate levels have two or three times the risk of having a baby with certain spinal cord problems. For this reason, supplemental folate is now added to grain products. Women who are not using contraception and still at risk of pregnancy should consider taking folic acid supplements in order to keep their overall daily folic acid intake at 400 micrograms per day. Intake at this level clearly reduces the risk of these congenital spinal cord problems.

Folic acid has also been studied for its possible use in reducing breast cancer. Increased folate intake has been linked to lower breast cancer risk in women who drink alcohol, probably because alcohol reduces the ability of the body to use folic acid. In women who don't drink, taking supplemental folic acid does not seem to decrease the risk of breast cancer.

Heart disease is a common killer of women, and taking B vitamins, particularly B_6 and B_{12}, may decrease the risk of heart disease, although this topic needs further study. Finally, vitamin E supplements may reduce the risk of Alzheimer's disease, although again, this needs further study.

Almost all studies of vitamin intake offer substantial evidence that vitamins found in food are much more useful than those taken as supplements. This should be an encouragement to eat a healthy diet high in vegetables, whole grains, and low-fat dairy products. If you are unable to modify your diet in this way, then taking supplemental calcium, vitamin D, folic acid, and possibly vitamin E may be useful.

FOODS THAT MAY HELP PAIN

Most women do not get enough calcium in their diets, and calcium is the primary mineral in bone. Low calcium intake is associated with greater menstrual pain, and calcium supplements have been shown to significantly reduce symptoms of PMS (premenstrual syndrome). Women should get 1,200 mg a day of calcium (1,500 mg if they are pregnant). An eight-ounce glass of milk or a one- to two-ounce serving of cheese has about 300 mg of calcium, so supplemental calcium may be a good idea unless you eat four servings of dairy products a day. Foods rich in calcium include kelp, cheese, almonds, and anchovies or sardines (the little bones are very high in calcium).

Calcium supplements come in many forms. Studies have shown that supplements containing calcium citrate are better absorbed than supplements made primarily of calcium carbonate or oyster shell calcium. Calcium citrate is, however, more expensive than other forms of calcium supplements.

Many antacids, such as Tums, Mylanta Lozenges, or Maalox

Antacid Caplets, are mostly calcium and a relatively inexpensive source of calcium carbonate. A typical antacid tablet contains approximately 300 mg of calcium. When taking calcium carbonate sources of calcium supplements, avoid consuming foods high in fiber or oxalates (tea) at the same time because they can bind with the calcium and actually decrease bodily absorption.

Calcium supplements should not be taken in doses greater than 500 mg at a time, as absorption generally does not occur in higher doses. So, if you take a calcium supplement be sure to take it several times throughout the day, each time taking no more than 300–500 mg.

Finally, calcium supplements are known to interact with or prevent the absorption of many medications. As a general rule, it is best to separate antacid use and any other medications by at least one hour. Although this list is not complete and you should always check with your physician and pharmacist to verify potential interactions with any medications you may be taking, the following are a few common medications known to interact with calcium supplements:

- Corticosteroids (prednisone, hydrocortisone, etc.)
- Digoxin (high levels of calcium may increase the likelihood of a toxic reaction when taken with digoxin)
- Loop diuretics (furosemide, torsemide, etc.)
- Thiazide diuretics (hydrochlorothizide, benzthiazide)
- Flecainide (Tambocor)
- Phenytoin type drugs (Dilantin, Mesantoin, Peganone, Cerebyx)
- Iron (calcium decreases iron absorption if taken at the same time)
- Quinidine (Quinidex, Quinaglute)
- Aspirin, salicylates

- Tetracycline (doxycycline, oxytetracycline)
- Ciprofloxain (Cipro)

NUTRIENTS: REPLACING ANIMAL PRODUCTS

Vegetarians who eat no animal products need to be more aware of nutrient sources. Some nonanimal sources of key nutrients are identified in the following table. In addition, nutrition counseling may help provide the guidance necessary for developing a nutritionally adequate vegetarian diet.

Nutrient	Vegetarian Replacement
Calcium	Almonds Anchovies Bok choy Broccoli Grain products Greens Kale Kelp Legumes (peas and beans) Lime-processed tortillas Nuts Orange juice (calcium enriched) Seeds Soy and rice beverages (calcium enriched) Tofu (processed with calcium)
Iron	Blackstrap molasses Brewer's yeast Cereals and breads (iron fortified) Dried fruit Green leafy vegetables Legumes Nuts Tofu Wheat germ Whole grains *Note:* Iron absorption is increased with vitamin C, found in

citrus fruits/juices, tomatoes, strawberries, broccoli, peppers, dark green leafy vegetables, and potatoes with skins.

Protein	Grains
	Legumes (kidney, lima, black, pinto beans; peas, chickpeas, black-eyed peas)
	Nuts
	Peanut butter
	Quinoa (gluten-free cereal)
	Seeds
	Seitan (meat substitute made from wheat gluten)
	Tempeh (meat substitute made from soybean, rice, and a grain culture)
	Tofu (curd of soybean milk)
	Vegetables (spinach, broccoli, potatoes)
Vitamin B$_{12}$	Cereals (fortified)
	Soy and rice beverages (fortified)
Vitamin D	Soy and rice beverages (fortified)
	Sunshine
Zinc	Legumes
	Nuts
	Tofu
	Whole grains
	Whole wheat bread

Source: National Uterine Fibroids Foundation.

Eating nutritiously may help you deal with fibroids both directly, by reducing symptoms, and indirectly, by increasing your overall health and maybe even reducing new fibroid growth over time. Eating a good, balanced diet high in fiber and low in fat may help you curtail bleeding and pain. Cutting down your consumption of beef, ham, and other red meat and dairy products while increasing your consumption of fish, whole grains, legumes, vegetables, fruits, and other non-processed foods may be a helpful adjunct to medical treatment. Most vitamin and mineral supplements have not been studied well enough to make us recommend them as a routine part of treatment for fibroids. Gaining vitamins and minerals from a healthy diet is far superior to trying to overcome a poor diet by taking pills. However, taking supplements in reasonable amounts has very little risk, so if you want to try it, feel free to do so. Another useful lifestyle change, exercise, is highlighted in the next chapter.

Chapter 7

Exercise

This chapter discusses the health benefits of exercise and, more specifically, how regular, vigorous exercise can help you deal with symptoms from fibroids. Always consider your own physical limitations, of course, and start any new exercise regimen gradually. Discussing an exercise program with your doctor may be unnecessary unless you have heart problems or other serious medical conditions. If you have heavy bleeding, however, it is a good idea to seek the guidance of your physician before starting an exercise program.

Exercise relieves physical, mental, and emotional stress, and it helps reduce anxiety and depression. Exercise helps control weight, and it often helps reduce pain. This chapter includes tips on choosing an appropriate exercise routine to help with symptoms of fibroids, as well as advice on using exercises to recover from surgery.

Exercise strengthens the heart, lungs, and mind and helps the body efficiently use food. Regular exercise slowly but surely burns fat and strengthens muscles. Exercise increases levels of pain-relieving endorphins. It provides additional oxygen to the brain and nervous system. It lowers levels of stress hormones such as cortisol. It reduces your risk of heart problems, cancer, and other major diseases. Exercise is so good for you that it's a wonder it's still free!

Here are some well-established general health benefits of exercise:

- Reduces stress
- Helps control weight
- Reduces muscle tension
- Improves mental functioning
- Improves mental outlook
- Improves sleep
- Helps combat depression
- Extends life expectancy
- Reduces heart attack risk
- Lowers blood pressure

All treatments for fibroids work best for women who are as healthy as possible, which means eating as nutritiously as possible and exercising regularly. If you are not exercising very much, beginning a program of regular exercise is the single best thing you can do for your health. Start a new exercise program slowly and increase it over time as you build up stamina.

For most women, we recommend regular, sustained physical activity for thirty minutes at a time at least four days a week. Stretching the muscles, whether done before or after exercise, increases muscle flexibility. This can improve posture and help prevent or relieve muscle pain.

Aerobic exercise in which your heart rate remains consistently elevated gives the heart and lungs a good workout. Swimming, walking, running, and bicycling are all aerobic activities. If the exercise is weight bearing, such as walking, weight lifting, and tennis, it can also help prevent osteoporosis. Any regular exercise can also help relieve the pain associated with fibroids or menstruation.

Exercise may even lower your risk of getting fibroids. A study conducted at the Harvard School of Public Health looked at the incidence of benign reproductive system tumors (mostly fibroids) in approximately five thousand women, about half of whom were former athletes and half of whom were not. The researchers at Harvard found that the women who were former athletes had fewer benign reproductive system tumors than did the women who were not athletes. The study concluded that nonathletes had a 45 percent greater risk of benign reproductive tumors than did athletes.

A 1993 study conducted in Poland examined risk factors for fibroids by comparing a group of seventy-two women with fibroids and another group of women without them. Researchers found that the women with fibroids were more overweight and engaged in less physical activity than the women without fibroids. The women with fibroids also had higher levels of mental stress, which can sometimes be relieved by exercise.

This lower risk of fibroids in athletic women may be because women who exercise have a lower level of overall body fat. Less fat translates into lower levels of estrogen in the bloodstream, since some of the body's estrogen is made in fat tissues, and lean bodies with less fat make less estrogen. In addition, women with very low fat levels may stop ovulating and have lower estrogen levels, which may put them at less risk for fibroids. Other studies have found that former athletes also have fewer breast cancers and cancers of the reproductive system, indicating that exercise correlates with a reduced risk of these hormone-dependent cancers as well. As with the diet studies, none of these studies suggested that exercise or weight loss gets rid of fibroids that are already there. Nonetheless, exercise is good for you and may retard the growth of new fibroids or reduce symptoms from fibroids you already have.

CONTROLLING PAIN

The most direct benefit of exercising regularly for women with fibroids is that it may help reduce levels of pain and menstrual cramps. Women with fibroids often involuntarily contract the muscles of the lower back or pelvis as a response to physical or emotional stress. Pain results as muscle tension decreases blood flow and oxygenation to the tense area. This slows down the movement of waste products such as lactic acid, which can cause pain, out of the area. Exercise makes your heart beat faster and increases your breathing. This increases blood circulation and the flow of oxygen to the uterine muscles. Using your muscles, as you do with exercise, reduces muscle tension all over the body. All of this helps reduce pain.

Exercise also increases the level of pain-relieving endorphins in the bloodstream, and these naturally reduce the sensation of pain. A 1985 study in the *Journal of the American College of Health* showed that women who were randomly assigned to exercise thirty minutes a day, three days a week, had significantly less menstrual pain than an equal number of women who were randomly assigned to be "couch potatoes."

Although it's not generally considered an aphrodisiac, exercise may also enhance your sex life. A study at the University of British Columbia in Vancouver, Canada, looked at thirty-five Canadian women, aged eighteen to thirty-four, who were all involved in heterosexual relationships prior to the study.

Blood flow to the vagina, or genital engorgement, an indicator of sexual arousal, was measured using *vaginal photoplethysmography*, which measures changes in blood flow to the vagina. Women in this study were asked to watch an erotic video—both without exercising and after a twenty-minute session on a stationary bicycle. When they watched the erotic video after they exercised, the women's genital engorgement increased 168 percent, even though they were not consciously aware of the physical change.

> One woman we know was having problems with sexual response after medical treatment for fibroids. The woman began exercising vigorously and routinely, primarily to get her strength back and to improve her mood. After a period of time, and to her great surprise, she found that exercising in this manner for five nights a week contributed to increased genital engorgement, sexual energy, and sexual response for several hours after she returned home from the gym.

Other research has shown that women who exercise regularly do not suffer from premenstrual syndrome (PMS) as often as women who do not exercise do. In one study conducted in Australia, 97 women who exercised regularly were compared to a group of 159 women who didn't exercise. Women who exercised had markedly better concentration, more ebullient moods, less behavior change, and less pain during their menstrual cycle.

In another study conducted in England, a group of women who exercised competitively, a group of women who exercised regularly, and a group of women who were sedentary were compared for symptoms of depression and anxiety during three phases of their menstrual cycles. Women who exercised the most were the least anxious and depressed and also seemed happier, further evidence that exercise can prevent some common mood problems.

CHOOSING AN EXERCISE

Exercise should be done almost every day for maximum benefit, but women who are mostly sedentary will get enormous benefit from as little as ten minutes a *week* of exercise. To help assure that you can keep it up, the exercise you select should fit your interests and lifestyle. Pick either one form of exercise or a cluster of activities that you enjoy that will keep you from getting bored. Some women like to concentrate on one thing and do it well; others like to mix it up with several different types of exercise each week.

If you're a social person, you may enjoy exercising with a friend, joining a sports club, dancing, or getting involved in team sports such as volleyball. If you prefer to exercise alone, you may enjoy running, skating, bicycling, or swimming. You may prefer a more leisurely form of exercise such as walking or gardening. If you haven't exercised in a while, think of the activities you used to enjoy and use that as a place to start selecting an exercise.

Walking is one of the safest and most natural forms of exercise, and we frequently recommend it as a gentle and low-cost way to start exercising. A good pair of walking shoes is about all you need to begin walking; some communities have mall-walking clubs if you like to exercise in a group, or if you need some cover during the winter. Hiking is a variation of this, very weather dependent, and a bit more strenuous, but it gives you some time in a more pristine and beautiful environment than most cities afford.

YOGA AS EXERCISE

One of the best forms of exercise that may benefit women with fibroids is yoga. Yoga is an ancient discipline combining stretching exercises with periods of relaxation and deep controlled breathing. Currently enjoying a surge in popularity, yoga has many health benefits: strengthening the body, calming the mind, and improving overall flexibility and balance. Yoga's emphasis on controlled breathing reduces stress; it is considered a stress-relieving mind/body therapy.

As a therapeutic exercise, yoga is best practiced in a class, where an instructor guides you through various postures. The instructor should assure important moments of deep relaxation and breathing between postures and help with fine points such as how to position the hands and feet. All this makes sessions more relaxing and useful. Yoga classes are available in most communities through schools, YMCAs, or recreation programs, often at a reasonable cost.

Pilates and Feldenkrais are two forms of exercise similar to yoga that contribute to posture control and gently stretch and strengthen the muscles. Other possibly beneficial forms of exercise include the ancient Chinese exercises tai chi and chi gong, which are quite gentle and have proven to be good for your heart and blood pressure.

EXERCISE AFTER SURGERY

Exercise is also a good way to help your body gain strength and recover from invasive treatments for fibroids. Exercising before surgery will help you build up your strength and stamina both for the surgery itself and for your recovery after the surgery. Surgery is a major stress on your body, and it will deplete your strength for a time. Lying in a hospital bed, even for only a day or two, causes muscles to become weaker. Most women aren't able to exercise at all for a few weeks after surgery because they are in some pain as tissues heal.

It is important to take it easy for a while when getting back into an exercise program after invasive procedures. Your body takes time to heal after surgery, and you can hurt yourself by getting too active too soon. In consultation with your medical doctor, begin your exercise sessions slowly after surgery. Use common sense. Exercise only for a short period of time at first, and then slowly build up your time in exercise sessions.

After you get home from the hospital, you'll probably be limited in your ability to exercise. You'll be taking pain medication and won't have much energy. Gradually, as your energy returns, you can increase your activity level. One of the best things to do as a way of getting back into exercise is to begin walking regularly. You can begin a week or so after surgery if you feel up to it just by walking up and down the street. You need to listen to your body and gradually increase the distance that you walk without hurting yourself. The way to do this is to walk farther than you did the previous day but not so far that you begin to hurt. Finding this balance can sometimes be difficult, but it's important not to overdo it when you're recovering because this can set you back even further. After you're able to walk for at least twenty minutes without resting, then you are probably ready to advance to more strenuous exercises.

You probably shouldn't begin doing any heavy lifting or weight training until at least several months after surgery, unless your doctor advises you otherwise. If you've had major abdominal surgery, such as a myomectomy, your abdominal wall is weakened by the surgery. Even though the skin may be healed, the strength of your abdominal wall is not fully restored for up to six months after surgery. This doesn't mean that you need to wait six months before doing any abdominal exercises or weight lifting, only that you need to begin these exercises gradually and give your body plenty of time to heal.

Three keys to returning to exercise after surgery are as follows:

- Discuss your exercise plan with your doctor.
- Begin slowly.
- Don't put any extra strain on your abdominal muscles until at least several months after surgery.

Exercise Possibilities

Column A lists extremely vigorous exercises.*
Column B lists moderately vigorous exercises.
Column C lists simply enjoyable, less vigorous activities.

Column A†	Column B	Column C
Basketball	Tai chi	Bowling
Cross-country skiing	Badminton	Camping
Bicycling	Weight lifting	Fishing
Gymnastics	Calisthenics	Gardening
Hiking	Dancing	Golfing
Jogging	Downhill skiing	Softball
Aerobics/Jazzercise	Walking	Volleyball
Wind surfing	Karate	Horseshoes

Skating		Chi gong	Table tennis
Soccer		Tennis	
Swimming			
Rowing		Feldenkrais/Pilates/yoga	
Water skiing			

*Whether an exercise is listed as extremely, moderately, or less vigorous often depends on the degree of effort made.

†Some exercises identified in this table require appropriate guidance from a certified trainer to develop proper form and avoid injury.

Chapter 8

Stress

Lifestyle changes that reduce stress give you a measure of control over fibroid symptoms. This chapter explains how stress affects many women with fibroids and presents some of the mind/body therapies such as biofeedback, deep breathing, and relaxation techniques that can help you deal with it effectively. In addition to helping you control symptoms, reducing stress can improve your overall health.

Women are under stress. We live in a dynamic, pressure-cooker society, and while society offers enormous material rewards for achievement, the downside of this pressure to achieve is stress. Problems with relationships, finances, careers, and more contribute to a generally high level of stress. Having a health problem such as fibroids adds even more stress. There is little research on the effects of stress on women with fibroids, but many doctors have heard women remark that their fibroids seem to grow faster when the women are under stress.

Stress can intensify pain or muscle tension, which can accumulate in areas such as the lower back, pelvis, stomach muscles, shoulders, and arms. Tension can be experienced as headache pain or a general fatigue. Fortunately, reducing stress releases this muscle tension. Reducing stress levels also helps normalize the timing of the release of important hormones.

Stress can disrupt chemical messages between glands such as the hypothalamus and pituitary, which regulate the menstrual cycle, and thereby trigger abnormal or excessive menstrual bleeding. The hypothalamus produces gonadotropin-releasing hormones (GnRH), and the pituitary gland releases follicle-stimulating and luteinizing hormones (FSH and LH). The closely timed release of these pituitary hormones helps regulate the menstrual cycle, and stress can alter this delicately balanced system.

Stress changes your body. When you experience acute stress, your body shifts into a "fight or flight" survival mode, which rapidly changes your body chemistry. Blood sugar rises, blood pressure shoots up, and stress hormones such as adrenaline and cortisol flood the body. Muscles tense up as a natural preparation to "fight or flee." It makes sense that these disturbances can affect symptoms of fibroids and that controlling stress can help relieve these symptoms.

RESEARCH ON STRESS AND FIBROIDS

Researchers have identified stress as an *associated* risk factor for women with fibroids, but there is no research that proves that stress actually *causes* fibroids. Furthermore, there is no consistent association between stress reduction and the prevention or resolution of fibroids. However, a few studies do seem to relate stress to fibroids.

Research in Poland found higher levels of stress biomarkers in fibroid tissues as opposed to normal uterine tissues. Women with larger fibroids also had higher levels of this chemical in their bodies. Other research has linked fibroids to high levels of anxiety. However, these studies were completed over a decade ago and have not been repeated or confirmed.

While some researchers have attempted to look at the effects of managing stress on uterine fibroids and symptoms, this research should not lead you to believe that fibroids are your "fault" or that you can control their growth by merely controlling your stress. Simply having and experiencing symptomatic fibroids can be stressful, so it's hard to know which came first—fibroids or stress. However, like increasing exercise, reducing stress is good for you, so stress reduction is certainly worth trying.

Most people are under so many different types of stress that their lives feel out of control. It can be useful to divide stressful things in your life into those you can control and those you cannot control. Simply recognizing that certain things are beyond your personal control can be helpful. For instance, it is beyond your control that you have been diagnosed with uterine fibroids. This is a simple fact. However, you have a great deal of control over choosing an appropriate medical treatment for yourself by working with your medical doctor to understand your treatment options. You cannot control that your doctor advises you to have a hysterectomy, but you do have the power to seek a second opinion and to research your medical options. You may not be able to control the fact that you have bleeding or pain, but you may be able to institute lifestyle changes that help you control these symptoms. In the larger arena of your life, minimizing your exposure to people or situations that you find personally stressful can help lower stress levels.

If you feel overwhelmed, you may want to see a therapist, psychologist, or psychiatrist who can help you sort through your problems and life issues. Support groups, either in-person meetings or on the Internet, are helpful to many women with health problems. Support groups typically bring together women with similar health concerns on a regular basis and give them a chance to discuss their health issues in a supportive environment.

MIND/BODY THERAPIES

Mind/body therapies are extremely gentle and can often complement other medical treatment. Some are best learned from professional therapists, but once learned, they may be used as needed at home. Others are closer to self-help techniques. In addition to yoga, covered in the previous chapter on exercise, relaxing mind/body therapies include aromatherapy, bodywork, breath control, progressive muscle relaxation, prayer, hypnosis, meditation, visual imagery, and even writing. Blood pressure, blood sugar, stress hormone levels, heart rate, and muscle tension are all reduced with the practice of mind/body therapies.

• *Aromatherapy* involves concentrated aromatic fragrances and scents that reportedly have a direct pathway to the brain. A few drops of essential oil may be added to bathwater or mixed with vegetable oils for a stress-relieving, aromatic massage. Select fragrances that appeal to you. Possibilities include stress-relieving lavender, one of the most popular. *Note:* Some women with high sensitivity to fragrances or floral scents may not tolerate aromatherapy. Always use your best judgment in applying any of the mind/body therapies listed in this section.

• *Bodywork.* Most people feel relaxed after being massaged. Massage works on the body's largest organ, the skin, to increase blood and lymph circulation in the body, which may reduce pain. Simply relaxing tensed muscles on a regular basis reduces pain and helps clear the mind. In one study of 138 women with painful menstruation, spinal manipulation showed some pain-relieving effect. Massage is an aspect of treating fibroids in other health systems such as Chinese and Ayurvedic medicine.

• *Breath control.* Most people under stress breathe too quickly, drawing breaths from the top of the lungs. Slowing your breath to perhaps four or five deep abdominal breaths per minute helps relax tense muscles in your body and slows your heartbeat as you also take in more oxygen. Breath control exercises can be done sitting up in a chair or lying down with your knees up. Imagine each inhalation filling your body with energy and each exhalation releasing tension and stress. In one study, menopausal women troubled by hot flashes reduced their intensity 40 percent over a twenty-four-hour period using controlled breathing, even when compared with women who used progressive muscle relaxation or biofeedback.

• *Progressive muscle relaxation* involves deep breathing and relaxing sets of muscles in a slow, rhythmic fashion. One study showed an improvement in some symptoms in women with spasmodic painful menstruation using either relaxation training or relaxation training plus visual imagery. Yet another study found that relaxation sessions twice a week for three months improved painful menstruation in high school girls.

• *Prayer* is a form of meditation that relieves stress for many people. Several studies have shown that people who participate regularly in religious services are healthier than people who do not; they have lower blood pressure and fewer heart attacks and generally live longer lives. A recent study of the power of prayer published in the *British Medical Journal* showed that prayer reduced fever in patients with infection—even when the praying was done by someone unknown to the patient. Similar studies have shown prayer to increase pregnancy rates in women having fertility problems.

• *Hypnosis* is a recognized therapy for pain control. Some therapists believe that bleeding may also be controlled through hypnosis, by visualizing the blood vessels of the uterus being squeezed shut. Autogenic therapy and affirmations are forms of self-hypnosis that may be very helpful in bolstering health. Many studies affirm the value of autogenic training.

• *Meditation* lowers stress; many studies show decreased levels of stress hormones such as cortisol during sessions of quiet meditation. Practicing meditation counteracts the physical effects of stress.

• *Visual imagery.* Although no studies specifically test this technique for treating fibroids, some naturopathic/alternative medicine physicians recommend visualization exercises along with a low-fat diet, regular aerobic exercise, and 400 IU of vitamin E twice a day as a treatment for women with fibroids.

• *Writing* about traumatic events relieves stress, according to several research studies. Keeping a journal can be helpful.

Stress affects your entire body, and it can intensify symptoms such as bleeding and pain. Fibroids can intensify physical and mental stress. Relieving stress through the regular practice of mind/body therapies can help you deal with fibroids. At the very least, finding ways to reduce stress can give you a feeling of control over your life. Lifestyle measures including diet and exercise may help you deal with fibroids too.

Controlling stress, improving your diet, and increasing your exercise level can help you improve your health and are among the safest lifestyle changes you can try. If these aren't enough, you may want to consider medical therapies or treatment. The next chapter begins an examination of alternative therapies that can be invaluable aids in controlling symptoms.

Chapter 9

Alternative Medicine

This chapter looks at alternative or complementary therapies of interest to many women. We include information on Western herbs, acupuncture, Asian herbal medicine, homeopathy, and some home remedies. We present these things because many women want to try them as part of a holistic approach to treating fibroids.

For the most part, alternative therapies have not been as well researched as pharmaceuticals, but many alternative therapies included here have been used for many years. We have had patients report that their fibroids shrank dramatically after starting one of these therapies, but we have also had patients whose fibroids actually *grew* when taking herbal treatments.

Remember: Anything strong enough to work is strong enough to be dangerous. Do not assume that "alternative" means safe. "Alternative" means that the treatment is outside the scope of most medical research. One danger of alternative therapies is that they might cause you to abandon proven medical treatments. We advise women with fibroids to keep their gynecologist apprised of any alternative treatment they use, and to have regular pelvic exams and ultrasound examinations to see if the therapy is having any positive or negative effect on their fibroids. We provide this list of alternative therapies as a description of what exists. The lack of scientific study of these things makes us unable to recommend most of them as standard treatments, just as we would not recommend surgery or traditional drugs if they had not been adequately tested.

Generally, alternative therapies are much slower to take effect than traditional drugs. Both nutritional and herbal approaches often take effect quite slowly, reducing symptoms only a little at a time. Herbal remedies for bleeding may take several weeks or months to have any appreciable effect. Tori Hudson, a naturopath specializing in women's health issues, suggests that women try nutritional or herbal treatments for a couple of hours for pain, but if they don't work, that they switch to a drug that does. After that, Dr. Hudson suggests that women try to gradually lengthen the time they allow nutritional or herbal treatments to work in subsequent episodes.

COMPLEMENTARY TREATMENT OF UTERINE FIBROIDS

The most thorough study to date of alternative treatments for fibroids shows that these treatments may be quite effective in relieving symptoms. Dr. Louis Mehl-Madrona studied seventy-four women with fibroids and treated half with a series of complementary methods. Most of the women had problems with bleeding, but some had pain, and a few had fatigue as their primary symptom. Each patient had an individually designed traditional Chinese medicine regimen. These treatment regimens included acupuncture, Chinese herbs, meditation, nutritional therapy, guided imagery, and pelvic bodywork. The women who received standard treatment were treated mostly with hormonal therapy and pain medication.

Overall, the number of women who had improvement was remarkably similar between the two groups. Nineteen out of forty women treated with traditional Chinese medicine and sixteen out of forty treated with traditional medicine improved at the end of six months.

Even though the two groups had nearly equivalent improvement, this study is dramatic because it is the most well designed study to examine nontraditional treatments for fibroids. Treatment was also very expensive with women in the nontraditional medicine group paying approximately $3,800 over the course of six months. Needless to say, these treatments are generally not covered by insurance.

Traditional Chinese medicine treatments are integrated in order to provide the best results for each patient, so there is no simple way to turn this study into a prescription for other women. It does suggest the value of alternative treatments. If you want to pursue complementary treatment for fibroids, try to find an experienced practitioner who has extensive formal training. Be wary of people who promise they can cure your fibroids, and be willing to give up or change treatments if you aren't seeing results.

TRADITIONAL CHINESE MEDICINE

Traditional Chinese medicine is a system that includes complicated herbal formulas as well as acupuncture and related therapies. In contrast to Western medicine, Asian medicine looks at fibroids as problems caused by "blood stagnation," in which the normal flow of energy and blood is disrupted, creating toxic solids such as fibroids in the body. A condition known as "empty blood" is said to lead to depression and menstrual problems. The *Nei Ching*, a classic medical text of China, states that a great grief, anxiety, or too much thinking—what we in the West might call excessive stress—can cause a tumor such as a fibroid.

Acupuncture involves the insertion of fine needles into points on the body along energy pathways, called meridians, which are believed to correspond to anatomical structures. One of these, the Chung Mo pathway, a special meridian located on the front of the body, is said to flow through the pelvic area and female reproductive organs. Acupuncture is widely accepted as a therapy to control many types of pain.

Acupuncture can be useful in treating pain arising from fibroids, menstrual pains, or endometriosis. A study published in the *American Journal of Chinese Medicine* used acupuncture on a group of forty-eight women with painful menstruation, with favorable responses in more than 58 percent of the women in the study, and satisfactory results in 25 percent. Approximately 8 percent of the women reported no relief. In a second study published in *Obstetrics and Gynecology*, ten of eleven women found pain relief with acupuncture, and 41 percent were able to reduce their use of pain medications.

Acupuncture for Fibroids

Dr. Dennis Kessler, a Los Angeles acupuncturist, says he has treated several women for pain who also had fibroids or ovarian cysts. Acupuncture treatments for pain often slowed the growth of fibroids, he said. Several patients subsequently had ultrasounds showing that their fibroids had shrunk, sometimes after only one acupuncture treatment. According to Dr. Kessler, acupuncture is often effective in reducing pain and is remarkably safe when performed by a licensed practitioner.

A study in the *British Medical Journal* found no serious complications out of more than 31,000 acupuncture visits. Minor complications, such as bleeding from the acupuncture site, happened in only 6 percent of cases.

Herbal formulations are another aspect of traditional Chinese medicine. Herbs are used differently in Asia—typically as mixtures of several herbs rather than one herb aimed at one symptom. A 1995 study published in the *Journal of Traditional Chinese Medicine* showed good results from the use of Chinese herbal formulations by a group of women with anovulatory dysfunctional uterine bleeding. The study included fifty-two women aged fourteen to fifty who received herbal decoctions; the formulations returned thirty-six of thirty-eight women who had not entered menopause back to normal periods. Rather than trying one drug, this study used a variety of herbal formulations to right the balance between energy polarities the Chinese call yin and yang.

Susan had severe bleeding from fibroids and was told by many doctors that she needed a hysterectomy. She looked for alternatives and found a Chinese herbal medicine practitioner who prescribed a mix of herbs for her. Initially, she found this treatment very effective, dramatically decreasing her bleeding for the first several months she took it. Eventually, the heavy bleeding recurred and she needed surgery. "I'm not sorry I tried the herbal treatment," said Susan. "Even though they weren't enough in the end, I went into surgery feeling that I had truly exhausted my other options, and that made me feel much more comfortable taking such a drastic step."

Japanese folk medicine uses herbal mixtures that may reduce pain. In one double-blind study of the effects of the Japanese *kampo* folk medicine Toki-shakuyaku-san (TSS) on forty women with painful periods, pain was significantly reduced in the group using the herbal remedy after two menstrual cycles, when compared with women in the placebo group. A mixture of six different herbs, TSS had no effect on the level of depression.

In another recent Japanese research study on women treated with GnRH agonists for fibroids, endometriosis, and adenomyosis, thirteen Japanese women with induced menopause experienced symptom relief of hot flashes and shoulder stiffness using *kampo* medicines. Estrogen levels were not adversely affected by the herbal mixtures.

WESTERN HERBAL MEDICINE

Herbal remedies are more widely used in Europe than in the United States. Proponents say that herbs are gentler than pharmacological drugs because they contain a natural mixture of chemical substances and produce fewer side effects. Western herbal medicine uses herbs in the same way medical doctors use drugs: A particular symptom is treated with a particular herb. Two reputable sources of information about medicinal herbs are the regularly updated reference book *Review of Natural Products* and *The Complete German Commission E Monographs*, a summary of research and recommendations on herbs conducted by doctors under the auspices of the German government. If you try herbal remedies, consult an experienced and competent practitioner. If you experience troubling side effects, stop taking the herb.

Stringent federal quality standards for prescription drugs

guarantee that when you fill a prescription, you get what you pay for. However, for supplements and herbs, which are classified as foods rather than medicines, strict government quality control doesn't exist, and you must rely on the integrity of the company that markets the products. Unfortunately, tests have shown that in more than one-third of these products, what's on the label is not what's in the bottle. Lesser or nonexistent quantities of herbs, as well as substances not listed on the label, have been frequently discovered.

If an herb is powerful enough to change the way your body works, it can cause side effects, and some women have had bad experiences with herbs. **Blue cohosh** or squaw root, for instance, was once recommended by many herbal practitioners and even celebrity doctor Andrew Weil for heavy bleeding caused by fibroids. Dr. Weil no longer recommends blue cohosh and cites a study printed in the *Journal of Natural Products* proving that blue cohosh causes birth defects in rats, producing embryos with nerve damage, twisted tails, and poor eye development. More troublesome, in a recent issue of the *Journal of Pediatrics,* a Seattle pediatrician reported that a woman who had taken blue cohosh while pregnant delivered a baby that had severe heart problems. The pediatrician carefully excluded other possible causes before concluding that blue cohosh caused the baby's heart problems.

Herbs for Bleeding

Among the many herbs sometimes recommended for abnormal bleeding are chaste tree, dong quai, ginger, red raspberry, and trillium.

Chaste tree or *Vitex agnus castus* has been used since the time of Hippocrates as a remedy for female problems, and to help regulate menstruation. The fruits of the tree, similar in appearance to peppercorns, were once thought to lower excessive libido in women. Free and conjugated progesterone has been found in the leaves and flowers; furthermore, chaste tree berries are said to stimulate the production of progesterone from the ovaries and help regulate menstrual cycles. In a recent study conducted in Germany, an extract of the fruit was found to significantly relieve depression, anxiety, craving, and hyperhydration caused by PMS. A standardized preparation of chaste tree is used to treat uterine bleeding in Germany, where herbal medicines are more commonly used than in the United States. Benefits of this herb can take three months to a year to become apparent. Side effects can include gastrointestinal reactions, itching, rashes, headaches, and increased menstrual flow.

Dong quai or angelica is seen as a "female" remedy in Asian medicine and is used to treat symptoms of menopause and excessive or painful bleeding. For dysmenorrhea, *The Encyclopedia of Natural Medicine* recommends that dong quai be started on day fourteen and continued until menstruation has stopped. Many women use dong quai to treat menopausal symptoms, although one recent study published in *Fertility and Sterility* showed no effect of this herb on symptoms or physical signs of menopause. Furthermore, dong quai acts as a blood thinner, so it absolutely must be stopped at least two weeks before any surgery.

Ginger has been used traditionally as an anti-inflammatory agent to reduce excessive menstrual blood flow. It may also have a positive effect on menstrual cramps since it has a relaxing effect on smooth muscle tissue such as the uterus.

Herbs for Bleeding

Herbs sometimes recommended by herbal practitioners for relief of excessive bleeding include the following:

- Chaste tree or *Vitex agnus castus*
- Cranesbill or *Geranium maculatum*
- Dong quai or *Angelica sinensis*
- Ginger or *Zingiber officinale*
- Goldenseal or *Hydrastis canadensis*
- Greater periwinkle or *Vinca major*
- Helonias or *Chamaelirium luteum*
- Horsetail or *Equisetum arvense*
- Lady's mantle or *Alchemilla vulgaris*
- Life root or *Senecio aureus*
- Mugwort or *Artemisia vulgaris*
- Pennyroyal or *Mentha pulegium*
- Savin or *Sabina officinalis*
- Shepherd's purse or *Capsella bursa pastorus*
- Squaw vine or *Mitchella repens*
- Yarrow or *Achillea millefolium*

Herbs for Pain

Among the herbs practitioners sometimes recommend for pain are black cohosh, crampbark, black haw, licorice root, white willow, and valerian.

Black cohosh (not to be confused with *blue cohosh*) or *Cimicifuga racemosa* roots and rhizomes are traditional herbal remedies for painful menstruation. American Indians also treated snakebite with it. Black cohosh is supposed to relax the uterus. Its actions are similar to estriol, the weakest form of estrogen; some women use it as an alternative to conventional hormone replacement therapy, according to the *Review of Nat-*

ural Products. A standardized extract called Remifemin has been used in Germany for fifty years to relieve cramps and help manage menopause. Black cohosh is said to reduce mood swings, anxiety, depression, as well as the pain and discomfort of menstrual cramps, a decline in libido, and vaginal dryness. Overdoses, however, may cause nausea, vomiting, dizziness, nerve or vision disturbances, slower pulse rate, or sweating. Black cohosh is not recommended for pregnant women since it may induce miscarriage or premature birth in large doses.

Herbs for Pain

Herbs sometimes recommended for pain include the following:

- Black cohosh or *Cimicifuga racemosa*
- Black haw or *Viburnum prunifolium*
- Crampbark or *Viburnum opulus*
- German chamomile or *Matricaria chamomilla*
- Ginger or *Zingiber officinale*
- Hops or *Humulus lupulus*
- Passionflower or *Passiflora incarnata*
- Helonias or *Chamaelirium luteum*
- Valerian or *Valeriana officinalis*
- Wild yam or *Dioscorea villosa*

Crampbark and **black haw** are medicinal herbs prescribed for chronic uterine and ovarian pains and menstrual cramps. Some studies show that both herbs relax uterine tissue. Some practitioners recommend crampbark when pains are spasmodic or congestive and radiate down the thighs. Black haw is usually preferred for pains that include heavy menstrual flow and for intermittent pains.

Licorice root, an Asian folk remedy for abdominal pain, is believed to lower estrogen and raise progesterone, and to block the adrenal hormone aldosterone, which contributes to water retention. Licorice in large and sustained doses can cause high blood pressure, so women with a history of hypertension, kidney failure, or diabetes, or women who use digitalis for heart problems should not use it.

White willow, from which aspirin is synthesized, has a long history of use for pain relief in both Chinese and Western medicine. It is sometimes prescribed to reduce menstrual cramps and related headaches as well as pain. As an herb, white willow has side effects similar to aspirin, including thinning the blood. It is extremely important to stop this medication at least two weeks in advance of any surgical procedures.

Valerian or *Valeriana officinalis* is a traditional treatment for anxiety and sleep disorders. Dr. Hudson suggests this herb for menstrual cramps and painful menstruation, although it can make you sleepy.

Herbs to Help the Liver

Herbs that support liver function may be helpful for women with fibroids since the liver breaks down estrogen and has many other important functions. A qualified practitioner such as a nutritionally oriented physician, a naturopath, or an experienced herbal practitioner should be consulted for the proper dose of herbal remedies for the liver.

Some herbalists suggest herbs such as *Chelidonium* or celandine, *Chionanthus* or fringe tree, dandelion root, or milk thistle on a daily basis to improve liver function. Indirectly, they say, these herbs may decrease bleeding. Yellow dock is believed to help the liver. Curcumin, or turmeric, which flavors many Indian dishes, also has liver-strengthening qualities, according to Dr. Susan Lark. Two other herbs that may strengthen the liver, yellow dock and pau d'arco, are also said to be good sources of nonheme iron.

Although they are not herbs, lipotropic factors, which reduce the amount of fat in the liver, are used by some alternative practitioners to improve liver function, according to Dr. Hudson. Pancreatic enzymes, which aid digestion, are also sometimes used as a supplement to treat bloating or to improve general health, but there is no research to support their use in women with fibroids. Indeed, taking enzymes by mouth, while a popular treatment for a variety of problems, probably has no effect on *anything* since these enzymes are broken down in the gastrointestinal tract long before they can exert any effect.

HOMEOPATHY

Homeopathy is a Western medical system developed by a German physician. It uses very dilute substances called *remedies* to stimulate what homeopathic practitioners call "the vital force," the body's ability to defend itself against chemical threats. These substances are diluted to the point where even the most sensitive test cannot find the original substance in homeopathic medicines. This means two things: There is no way to know if what you are buying is what it purports to be, and there is no known mechanism or theory that explains why homeopathy should work. You will probably not harm yourself using homeopathic remedies, but expecting them to actually affect fibroids may be hoping for too much.

Classical homeopathy involves a lengthy, in-depth interview focusing on not only physical symptoms, but also mental and psychological factors, after which the practitioner attempts to match all your symptoms with a particular homeopathic remedy. Remedies bolster overall health, or address particular symptoms such as fibroids, and should always be taken at the strength and frequency directed by a practitioner. Qualified homeopathic practitioners may be found by contacting the National Center for Homeopathy in Alexandria, Virginia.

According to the *Illustrated Encyclopedia of Natural Remedies*, among the homeopathic remedies that may help with menstrual problems is *Ipecac*, which may be useful for heavy bleeding with bright red blood, accompanied by nausea. *Sabina* may be useful for pain and bleeding including dark red blood containing clots. *Sepia* may be useful for an intense, bearing-down type of pain. *Colocynthis* may be useful for a cramping pain improved by pressure, and *Chamomilla* may relieve pain similar to labor pains.

Schuessler biochemic tissue salts, included in the homeopathic *materia medica*, may be purchased at health food stores and are easily self-administered. Developed by a German homeopath, they are keyed to the idea that disease is a result of an imbalance in mineral salts. *Bach Flower Remedies*, developed by an English homeopath, are very dilute floral dew essences said to relieve various types of emotional pain; these remedies also may be self-administered.

NATURAL PROGESTERONE

Home Comfort Remedies

Castor oil packs may reduce abdominal pain and relieve stress. To make a castor oil pack, place a piece of flannel, about twelve by fourteen inches across and several layers thick, over the abdomen. Pour on enough castor oil to wet the cloth, cover with plastic and a towel (and perhaps a heating pad), and leave in place for about an hour and a half. Some women sleep with a castor oil pack. The skin becomes soft, and excess castor oil may be cleaned with a little baking soda added to water. Place the castor oil pack in a plastic bag for reuse.

Heating pads are another safe, time-tested method for relieving pain. Use either a hot water bottle or an electric heating pad placed over the lower abdomen. A recent scientific study supported the idea that this simple treatment can reduce the need for pain medication in women with pelvic pain. Avoid placing the heating pad directly on the skin or sleeping with the heating pad, as a burn may result.

Warm baths or soaking in a *hot tub* or *Jacuzzi* may also provide some relief from pain as well as reduce stress.

Progesterone, in natural form, is sometimes recommended as a way to counter estrogen's stimulation of fibroid growth. A leading proponent of this approach, Dr. John Lee, author of the book *What Your Doctor May* Not *Tell You about Menopause*, believes that the use of natural progesterone will stop the growth of fibroids or cause them to shrink until menopause when fibroids naturally recede. Dr. Lee believes that uterine fibroids result from the "dominance" of estrogen over its complementary hormone, progesterone. Unfortunately, research has shown that this simple "estrogen bad, progesterone good" theory is far too simple and does not adequately explain the behavior of fibroids. Dr. Mitchell Rein, in a 1995 issue of *American Journal of Obstetrics and Gynecology*, cited biochemical and clinical evidence showing that progesterone actually promotes fibroid growth.

Dr. Lee believes that natural progesterone is significantly different from the artificial, chemically altered forms of progesterone called *progestins* used in most hormone replacement therapy and in birth control pills. He strongly believes that the effects of natural progesterone can help shrink fibroids, although we found no published studies confirming his theory.

Questions to Ask an Alternative Practitioner

- Where did you learn this therapy and how much training do you have in using it?
- Do you know of any research indicating that this treatment can affect uterine fibroids?
- How will I know if this therapy is working?
- How long, and at what frequency or dose, should I continue the treatments?
- What are the potential side effects, and how can I deal with them if they occur?
- What kind of results can I expect from this treatment?

Chapter 10

Drug Treatments

Medical therapies, including prescription and nonprescription therapies, are often useful in the treatment of fibroids. Several drugs can effectively help control bleeding and pain. Some drugs actually shrink fibroids, but these drugs may be dangerous when used for more than a few months. This chapter surveys the medications you may be able to use in the battle against fibroids, including some medications currently still considered experimental. It explains how they are properly used and their expected benefits and lists precautions and possible side effects. Hormonal medications require caution when used by women of childbearing age since some, such as Lupron, cause birth defects.

In Western medicine, drugs and surgery are the two most common methods of treating most diseases. In almost every case, doctors prefer drugs over surgery because the risks are generally lower. For some conditions, surgery may be more beneficial than drugs, but doctors don't usually decide this unless well-designed studies have proven the point. The reason is simple: Surgery is usually more dangerous. In some cases, surgery can relieve symptoms better than medications can for women with fibroids, but usually the dangers are greater as well. The results of taking medications are usually reversible, whereas surgery isn't. For these reasons, your doctor should generally recommend that you try medications before having surgery.

In our study of women who were inappropriately told that they needed a hysterectomy (discussed in more detail in chapter 1), one of the biggest mistakes doctors made in treating fibroids and many other conditions was not offering medications to their patients before recommending surgery. If your doctor recommends that you try some medications to treat the symptoms of your fibroids, and the medications don't work, you haven't lost much. You might spend a few weeks or even months trying the medication, but otherwise you're probably no worse off than you were when you started. If you have surgery and have a complication, however, you might have to live with the results of that complication for the rest of your life. Surgery is certainly the right thing to do in many circumstances, but it certainly makes sense to try less invasive therapies first.

MEDICAL THERAPIES THAT CONTROL SYMPTOMS

Medications work well enough for some women that they can live with their fibroids without ever needing surgery. Pain and bleeding can often be controlled with pain-relieving drugs, oral contraceptives, or other hormones, or sometimes a combination of medications.

One of the best studies of medication use to treat fibroids was called the Maine Women's Health Study. This study of 380 women found that medications significantly reduced symptoms from fibroids in most women. Women taking medications to treat bleeding had significant reductions in the number of days with bleeding. Women treated for pelvic pain achieved significant reductions in the number of days they experienced pain, and reductions in how much the pain bothered them.

Not all women in the study got relief from their problems, however. Even after medical treatment, about one-fourth of women who had abnormal bleeding continued to regard the bleeding as a problem, as did half the women with pelvic pain. About 10 percent of women treated with medications developed new symptoms including tiredness, hot flashes, weight gain, and depression. So medications aren't perfect. In the Maine study, approximately eight out of ten women who began using medical treatment for fibroids did not need any further treatment during the course of the study, while the remainder went on to need surgery. While what happened to these women may not exactly predict what will happen to you, it certainly is good news that the majority treated their fibroids without surgery!

Nonsteroidal Anti-Inflammatory Drugs (NSAIDs)

One of the most commonly used groups of drugs for fibroid pain is the nonsteroidal anti-inflammatory drugs (NSAIDs). This long name simply means that these medications work by reducing inflammation ("anti-inflammatory") and that they are not steroids ("nonsteroidal"). NSAIDs such as aspirin or ibuprofen are among the best first-line drug treatments for women with heavy menstrual flow, menstrual cramps, pain in the pelvis, or pressure in the abdominal region. These drugs have been studied for years, are reasonably safe, and clearly work to treat the symptoms of fibroids. NSAIDs are usually given to reduce pain, but they often decrease bleeding as well. The benefit of NSAIDs may be even greater when combined with oral contraceptives.

Some NSAIDs such as ibuprofen (Advil and Motrin are brand names of this drug) are available over the counter in the United States. One NSAID called mefenamic acid (Ponstel) may control pain and bleeding even better than ibuprofen, but it is available only by prescription. Using NSAIDs during the time of excessive bleeding reduces blood loss by 20 to 50 percent. To reduce excessive blood flow, typical doses are 600 milligrams of ibuprofen every six hours, 250 mg of mefenamic acid every six hours, or 550 mg of naproxen (Naprosyn) once a day. For best results, these drugs should be taken every day of the menses.

Using NSAIDs on a regular schedule can reduce inflammation and counteract pain. They do this by reducing a chemical called prostaglandin, present in high quantities in menstrual blood. Prostaglandin stimulates uterine contractions and causes pain.

There can be problems with these common drugs. About 10 percent of women who use them have digestive problems such as heartburn, nausea, diarrhea, constipation, or gastrointestinal bleeding. Taking the medications with food reduces these side effects. NSAIDs are often used as a first-line treatment of pain with strong painkilling drugs, including narcotics (drugs that are like morphine in their chemical action), used if the NSAIDs don't work. Long-term use of NSAIDs may increase the risk of gastrointestinal problems, kidney problems, and high blood pressure, but these risks must be weighed against the risks of other treatments, such as surgery or uterine fibroid embolization.

Birth Control Pills

> Kathy, a dental hygienist and long-distance swimmer, fought the pain of fibroids for many years with painkillers. Although her gynecologist frequently urged her to try birth control pills, she was fearful of disturbing her hormone levels with contraceptives. Finally, Kathy bit the bullet and went on the pill, and now she's glad she did. "It was such a relief," she says. "Now I'm off those painkillers." In Kathy's case, birth control pills adequately controlled the pain, making further treatment unnecessary.

Oral contraceptives can be highly successful in controlling bleeding from fibroids. Menstruation without ovulation, called *anovulatory* bleeding, common among women who are approaching menopause, is often controlled with birth control pills. Birth control pills may also be helpful for midcycle pain called *mittelschmerz.*

Birth control pills contain female hormones that stabilize the endometrium, the part of the uterus that bleeds, thereby stopping further hemorrhage. Studies of women with heavy bleeding found that oral contraceptives reduced blood loss about the same as NSAIDs. The pills even worked as well as stronger drugs, such as Danazol, which can have many more side effects. Low-dose oral contraceptives decrease blood loss by an average of 30 to 50 percent in most women, but results may be less impressive in women with fibroids.

For acute, very heavy bleeding, your doctor may suggest taking as many as four pills a day. This high dose cannot be used for long. However, if used for several days, it sometimes keeps serious bleeding from getting out of control. Since taking high doses of these pills often causes nausea, antinausea medications are often prescribed simultaneously.

Doctors usually prescribe birth control pills in cyclic fashion, meaning one pill is taken every day with a one-week break taken every month. Newer studies show that it is safe to skip the pill-free week for months at a time, moving from the active pills in one pack to the active pills in the next pack (skipping the last week of the pack because those are just sugar pills). This method, called continuous pill use, usually lessens menstrual flow even more than the usual way of taking the pills.

Birth control pills contain hormones that may affect the growth of fibroids. A few studies have found that oral contraceptives have a protective effect against fibroids, although other studies have not. Since fibroids and birth control pills are both quite common, it is surprising that more studies have not been conducted on the relationship between them.

If you do take birth control pills, it's a good idea to visit your gynecologist three months after starting the pills to have the size of your fibroids checked. Some doctors advise women with fibroids *not* to use birth control pills, but we disagree with this advice. The weight of the evidence suggests that taking birth control pills does not enlarge fibroids and *does* improve symptoms. If you are worried, have an ultrasound done before you start the pills and after three months to see if any change occurs. Women with high blood pressure or liver or gallbladder disease, women who have had breast or uterine cancer, smokers, or women with blood clots in their legs or pelvis may have additional risks from taking birth control pills and should discuss these risks with their doctors before taking them.

Progestins

Both medroxyprogesterone acetate (Provera) and megestrol acetate (Megace) contain a synthetic form of estrogen's complementary hormone, progesterone. Neither is labeled specifically for use in the treatment of fibroids, but they can be used to treat abnormal bleeding associated with fibroids. Provera is typically started in 10-milligram doses ten days before menses and continued every month for several months; however, studies have failed to show significant benefit from this regimen. Taking 10 mg per day for twenty-one days appears to be more effective, but does tend to produce side effects such as breast tenderness and bloating. Higher doses of 30 mg per day may be used temporarily to control bleeding. When control is achieved, the dose is tapered back to 10 mg a day for ten days.

Another progestin, *Depo-Provera* is a long-term contraceptive that may inhibit the development of fibroids. The prefix *depo* just means that the drug is stored in the body and released over time. A 1995 study published in the *British Journal of Obstetrics and Gynecology* found that women who used Depo-Provera for birth control had a lower risk of fibroids. The longer this contraceptive was used, the lower was the risk of fibroids. The benefits lasted as long as ten years after use— meaning that women who used Depo-Provera in their thirties had a lower risk of fibroids in their forties.

Because of studies like this, a number of gynecologists have given their patients with fibroids Depo-Provera, hoping it would shrink the fibroids. This doesn't seem like a good idea to us for several reasons. First, the studies linking Depo-Provera with lower risk of fibroids are *associational studies;* that is, Depo-Provera is only *associated* with fewer fibroids. This association doesn't mean that Depo-Provera actually prevents fibroids. It may be that women with fibroids are steered away from certain birth control methods (IUDs, for example, because they can be harder to use in women with fibroids) and toward Depo-Provera. This would make it seem as though the drug prevented fibroids, when in fact it didn't. Furthermore, these studies relate the development of fibroids with use of the drug; none of them showed the drug to shrink existing fibroids.

There is some reason to believe that treatment with progesterone-containing agents might have an *adverse* effect on fibroids. In particular, two studies used Provera pills in conjunction with another type of drug that usually shrinks fibroids, called a GnRH analog (described in more detail later). These studies found that when Provera was given with the GnRH analog, the GnRH analog no longer produced a reduction in fibroid size. In other words, adding Provera *prevented* the normal fibroid shrinkage that the other drug was causing. Research on Provera gives a mixed message, but generally supports the idea that both progesterone *and* estrogen are involved in fibroid growth.

If you have fibroids and need birth control, trying Depo-Provera should be fine, but it doesn't seem likely that it will melt your fibroids away. If you do start on this drug, having ultrasound exams several months apart will pick up any changes in fibroid size.

Tranexamic Acid

Tranexamic acid (Cyklokapron) is a drug known as an antifibrinolytic—a substance that prevents blood clots from dissolving. It is currently approved for use in the United States for treating individuals with bleeding disorders such as hemophilia or von Willebrand's disease. This drug has been tested in at least two randomized trials and found to significantly reduce menstrual blood flow. These studies show that tranexamic acid works better than Provera and NSAIDs in reducing abnormal or heavy bleeding. It seems to have few significant side effects, although about one-third of women taking it report having nausea and leg cramps. Because tranexamic acid increases blood clotting, there was initially some concern that it would increase the risk of dangerous blood clots (for example, clots that form in the legs and travel to the brains or lungs), but this risk does not seem to have been borne out in actual use. Tranexamic acid is typically taken only during the days of heavy menstrual flow.

Progestin-Releasing IUD

An intrauterine device or IUD that releases progestin is being used quite effectively in many countries to control bleeding, although is it not commonly used in the United States. Two studies of progestin-releasing IUDs have reported reductions in bleeding of up to 90 percent.

> **Jane suffered from heavy bleeding from fibroids. She was treated in a doctor's office with a hormone-releasing IUD. Within two weeks, Jane's bleeding stopped, thanks to a procedure about as painful as a menstrual cramp. Her bleeding is now under control.**

A study of 236 Finnish women with excessive bleeding published in the *Lancet* in 2001 compared women treated with either IUDs or hysterectomies. The study found IUDs successful in decreasing menstrual blood loss in most women. About three-fourths of the women had an easy insertion, and of the remaining 25 percent, most had only minor difficulties with placing the IUD. About one-third of the IUDs were removed in the first year because of side effects or lack of effect on bleeding. Many women had minor amounts of bleeding after insertion, but this usually resolved within three to six months. The success rate of hysterectomy at controlling bleeding was 100 percent. The IUD successfully controlled bleeding in 68 percent of women, but the remainder went on to have hysterectomies. For the women whose bleeding was well controlled by the IUD, it certainly must have seemed miraculous—a five-minute office procedure that improved their quality of life as much as a hysterectomy.

There is one progestin-releasing IUD on the market in the United States. The Mirena IUD releases Levo-Norgestrel (LNG), a type of progestin found to decrease heavy menstrual bleeding. Mirena may be left in place for up to five years. IUDs have not been widely used in the United States because of the bad experience of physicians with the Dalkon Shield, an IUD that was taken off the market in 1975. The Dalkon Shield caused pelvic infections, infertility, and even death but the design of that IUD, not IUDs in general, was the real problem. The Mirena IUD is very safe and has very few reported side effects.

Women using a progestin-releasing IUD tend to develop fewer fibroids than those who use other types of IUDs, according to a 1994 study by Irving Sivin published in the medical journal *Fertility and Sterility*. Women with preexisting fibroids were excluded from the study. Over the course of about eight years, fourteen of several hundred women using non-hormone-releasing IUDs developed fibroids, but none of the women who used progestin-releasing IUDs developed them.

At this time, there is not sufficient information to suggest that women who want to prevent fibroids begin using hormonal IUDs. However, because hormone-containing IUDs do tend to decrease menstrual bleeding dramatically, it may be a good idea for women with heavy bleeding to try this low-cost method. Placing an IUD in women with fibroids may be difficult, so you need to see a doctor who is experienced in inserting IUDs into all shapes and sizes of uteri.

MEDICAL THERAPIES THAT SHRINK FIBROIDS

A few drugs can shrink fibroids, but their effects stop when you discontinue the drugs. These drugs work by altering the levels of the body's normal hormones. The most commonly used are gonadotropin-releasing hormones or GnRH agonists, such as Lupron. Other drugs used to shrink fibroids include hormone antagonists and receptor blockers, synthetic steroids, interferon, and selective estrogen receptor modulators. Many of these drugs are experimental and should not be given to you unless you are enrolled in a study.

> One woman in her early forties recalls being put on Lupron, a GnRH agonist, for three months prior to surgery for fibroid-related bleeding. "When I went on Lupron, my periods stopped, and I had some spotting after that," she recalls. "I did pretty well at first. I didn't have any mood swings, but I had tremendous hot flashes. After that I was put on a progestin, and that took care of the hot flashes." In the final analysis,

she says, the drugs did their job of controlling bleeding and shrank the fibroids before surgery, when her doctor removed them.

Gonadotropin-Releasing Hormone (GnRH)

Gonadotropin-releasing hormone or GnRH is a hormone that regulates the menstrual cycle. GnRH fits into a special spot on the ovary, like a key into a lock. Natural GnRH in the body triggers the release of estrogen and progesterone from the ovaries, leading to ovulation and ultimately a menstrual period. Natural gonadotropin-releasing hormones have a half-life of only a few minutes, meaning that they break down very quickly and their effects last only a few minutes. However, the group of drugs called GnRH agonists (*agonist* means "acting like") is as much as two hundred times more potent than natural GnRH, and they remain much longer in the bloodstream. Natural GnRH is released in short bursts, with hundreds of bursts occurring over the course of a day. Artificial GnRH (which is what GnRH agonists are) fits into the same "lock" as natural GnRH, preventing the natural GnRH from getting where it is supposed to go. Without the normal GnRH bursts, the ovaries stop producing estrogen and progesterone, causing menstrual periods to stop temporarily.

The Lupron Scandal

Not long ago, a scandal enveloped Lupron's prime researcher, Dr. Andrew J. Friedman, a Harvard Medical School gynecologist, who falsified data in studies involving Lupron. Dr. Friedman's studies were published in two leading medical journals in 1993 and 1995, and retractions had to be printed. Dr. Friedman's medical license was suspended because of these disclosures. Unfortunately doctors still rely on several dozen of Dr. Friedman's studies when making clinical treatment decisions.

This episode is a small part of a much larger problem. Research on drugs is very expensive, and drug companies research their own products by paying individual doctors to recruit patients for studies. The doctors or their institutions are often paid for every patient they sign up, producing an obvious conflict of interest. The temptation to phony up data or design studies that will produce favorable results is obvious. Certainly, Dr. Friedman's falsified results cast a shadow on Lupron use for fibroids.

Because fibroid growth is dependent, at least in part, on estrogen, GnRH agonists also cause fibroids to shrink in most women. For unknown reasons, fibroids in some women don't respond to these drugs, while in a few others fibroids shrink almost completely.

GnRH agonists usually begin to work within two weeks. After about three months of treatment, shrinkage of fibroids peaks, with a typical reduction in uterine size of about 30 to 50 percent. Unfortunately, fibroids return to their original size about three months after medication is stopped. Periods return one to three months after stopping the drug. Generally speaking, women who are overweight show less reduction in uterine volume and may need higher Lupron doses. Doctors also believe that calcified tissue or more fibrous tissue in certain fibroids may be resistant to these drugs' effects. Continuing to take the medication will keep the fibroids at this reduced size, but they don't shrink much further even if drugs are continued for more than three months. Because GnRH agonists prevent normal estrogen production, continued use leads to osteoporosis and theoretically may raise the risk of heart attack, which is why these drugs are only good for short-term use.

GnRH agonists include leuprolide, nafarelin, and goserelin, which are sold under the brand names Lupron, Synarel, and Zoladex. Since GnRH is destroyed in the digestive system, GnRH agonists can't be taken in pill form or the hormone would just be inactivated in the stomach. Lupron is usually injected at the doctor's office, with one injection of Depo-Lupron usually good for a month; a three-month injection is also available. Zoladex is also injectible, but Synarel is a self-administered nasal spray, usually used twice a day, with the drug absorbed by the thin tissues of the nasal cavity.

There are pluses and minuses to each method of administration. Injected drugs must be given in the doctor's office, and their effects continue for a month or two even after the drug is stopped. Since Synarel is self-administered every day at home, it is less convenient, but it allows for a great deal of control. Synarel can be stopped at any time, and its effects usually wear off within two weeks. About one woman in ten develops a nasal irritation called *rhinitis* and must stop the medication.

Although gonadotropin-releasing hormone agonists can be used to shrink fibroids, the main use of these drugs is to stop periods so an anemic woman can regain a normal blood count. During a normal menstrual period a woman loses less than 80 cc (approximately five tablespoons) of blood, and her body easily makes up this amount before the next period. In women with fibroids or other causes for abnormal bleeding, the menstrual bleeding often outstrips the body's ability to keep up. The result is anemia. While this anemia is usually mild and can often be treated just by giving additional iron, which speeds the production of new red blood cells, sometimes it is important to treat anemia more aggressively.

If you become so anemic that your doctor worries that you might suffer additional health problems from it (being anemic puts additional strain on your heart), he or she might recommend treatment with a GnRH agonist. Because these agonists break the normal hormonal cycle, they prevent normal periods. Even in women who have bleeding unrelated to normal periods—such as the bleeding that sometimes accompanies fibroids—these drugs will often stop or dramatically reduce the bleeding. If you are anemic and facing surgery, then reducing your bleeding can be a tremendous benefit. This will allow your body to recover its normal blood count, possibly preventing or reducing the need for a blood transfusion.

GnRH agonists used before surgery may shrink fibroids to a more manageable size and may minimize the size of the incision needed for surgery. However, operative results are not always improved by the use of these drugs, as smaller fibroids may shrink so much that the surgeon misses them and they subsequently regrow.

GnRH agonists are also sometimes tried as a "holding action" to keep fibroids under control until menopause. This strategy only makes sense if you and your doctor believe you will be entering menopause within the next six months or so since fibroids quickly regrow after the drugs are stopped.

The most common side effects of GnRH agonists are the side effects of menopause, which are usually easy to control. Most women who use these drugs have hot flashes within the first month or so of treatment. Other side effects include lower sex drive, vaginal dryness, depression, weight gain, as well as loss of calcium and other minerals from the bones. Infrequent side effects occurring in 5 to 10 percent of patients include headache, insomnia, painful intercourse, weight loss or gain, muscle pain, hair loss, and swelling of the feet and ankles. The usual treatment for these symptoms is taking a synthetic progesterone substitute, such as norethindrone, or a small amount of estrogen, such as Premarin.

The loss of bone minerals or osteoporosis that occurs after prolonged use of GnRH agonists is a great concern. For this reason, doctors who prescribe GnRH agonists for longer than three to six months usually put their patients on hormone replacement therapy (HRT). HRT adds back estrogen (and sometimes progesterone) at low doses and helps prevent osteoporosis. Since long-term effects of prolonged GnRH therapy on overall health are unknown, we generally do not recommend this approach.

Irregular light vaginal bleeding occurs in 15 to 20 percent of patients taking GnRH agonists. Many women experience an episode of menstrual bleeding two days to two weeks after starting GnRH agonists, although periods typically stop after that. Although the drugs stop most heavy bleeding, an estimated 30 percent of patients continue to experience light intermittent bleeding, and a few continue to have heavy bleeding.

FDA-Approved Medical Therapies

Therapy	Names	Risks	Benefits
Nonsteroidal anti-inflammatory drugs (NSAIDs)	Aspirin Ibuprofen (Advil, Motrin, etc.) Mefenamic acid (Ponstel) Naproxen (Naprosyn)	Long-term use may cause gastrointestinal problems such as heartburn or bleeding and may bring on kidney problems and increased blood pressure.	Control heavy menstrual flow, menstrual cramps, and pelvic pain.
Birth control pills	Wide range	Increased risk of heart attack in smokers, increased risk of blood clots in legs.	Regulate menstrual cycle bleeding and may control abnormal bleeding.
Progestins	Medroxyprogesterone acetate (Provera) Megestrol acetate (Megrace)	Breast tenderness, bloating, weight gain.	May help to control bleeding.

Gonadotropin-releasing hormone agonists	Leuprolide acetate (Lupron) Nafarelin acetate (Synarel) Goserelin acetate (Zoladex)	Menopausal symptoms, osteoporosis, lower sex drive, vaginal dryness, depression, weight gain.	May control bleeding and shrink fibroids.
Tranexamic acid	Cyklokapron	Nausea and leg cramps.	Controls bleeding.
Hormone-releasing IUD	Progestin-releasing IUD (Mirena)	May be difficult to insert.	Reduces bleeding and may prevent new fibroids.

Mifepristone (RU-486)

Mifepristone, also known as RU-486, is a synthetic steroid hormone that suppresses progesterone and glucocorticoids. Mifepristone, currently sold under the brand name Mifeprex, is approved for use as a drug that causes abortion in early pregnancy—the so-called abortion pill. It causes abortion by blocking the effects of progesterone, which the body needs to support a developing pregnancy. Since this drug blocks progesterone, and fibroids seem to need progesterone to grow, it makes sense that taking it might cause fibroids to shrink. It is part of a class of "designer hormones," or hormone-like substances, that includes Tamoxifen and Raloxifene, which are described later.

Small pilot studies with mifepristone have shown good initial results at decreasing uterine blood flow and shrinking fibroids, about equal to GnRH agonists. In one study, conducted at the University of California at San Diego, women with fibroids who had regular menstrual cycles took 50 milligrams of mifepristone every day for three months. These women stopped having periods, and their fibroids decreased by almost 50 percent in volume. A major advantage mifepristone showed in this study over GnRH agonists was that sufficient levels of estrogen remained in the body to prevent osteoporosis.

In a second study of mifepristone, the same researchers reported that a dose of 25 mg per day achieved about the same size reduction as 50 mg per day, while a very small dose of 5 mg per day shrank fibroids 30 percent after three months. With both lower doses, all women in the trial stopped menstruating. Levels of progesterone in the bloodstream were reduced with all doses. Recent studies at Rochester University in New York have mimicked these results, and long-term studies are now in development using low daily doses of mifepristone. Remember the idea that estrogen was to blame for fibroid growth? The success of mifepristone certainly suggests that this is far too simple an explanation since its primary action seems to be blocking progesterone, not estrogen.

While mifepristone produces significantly fewer side effects than GnRH agonists, side effects do still occur. Some patients have hot flashes during the first month of treatment, and a few have had a temporary increase in joint pain. However, no long-term studies have been conducted on mifepristone, and fibroids do grow back after the drug is stopped, just as they do with GnRH agonists.

If mifepristone were to be used to treat fibroids over the long run, it would have to be taken every day, like a drug for high blood pressure or diabetes. At this point in time, and even though these short-term studies are exciting, too many things remain to be discovered about mifepristone's long-term effects for it to be a reasonable drug to use for treating fibroids. Hormone replacement therapy and birth control pills were studied for decades before their links with cancer and blood clots were identified. Unless long-term studies of mifepristone confirm its safety we cannot recommend it as a treatment for fibroids at this time.

Raloxifene and Tamoxifen

Raloxifene and tamoxifen are called selective estrogen receptor modulators (SERMs). These drugs are "designer drugs" specifically made to affect the body in ways similar to but not exactly the same as estrogen. Tamoxifen has been used for years to treat breast cancer since many breast cancers are sensitive to estrogen and tamoxifen blocks estrogen's effect on breast tissue. Tamoxifen has also been used to prevent breast cancer from starting in women who are at high risk. These drugs are called "selective" estrogen receptor modulators because they don't affect all tissues the same way. For example, tamoxifen, which blocks the effect of estrogen in the breasts, seems to act just like estrogen in the uterus. That is, the uterus responds to tamoxifen the same way it responds to estrogen. Specifically, women who take tamoxifen have a higher risk of developing endometrial hyperplasia (and even endometrial cancer). Sometimes that also happens to women who take estrogen.

Most of the information about the effects of tamoxifen on fibroids comes from studies of women who took tamoxifen to treat or prevent breast cancer. In a study published in the *Journal of Ultrasound Medicine*, seventeen postmenopausal women were treated with tamoxifen for breast cancer. Thirteen of the women had at least one fibroid, and during the course of treatment, six of the women developed new fibroids. The women did not develop symptoms from these fibroids, but the overall size of the fibroids did seem to increase. This study may no apply to all women but does suggest that tamoxifen is unlikely to be a good treatment for fibroids.

Raloxifene, like tamoxifen, is a SERM and has been used mostly in postmenopausal women. Its primary use has been to help prevent and treat bone loss since it acts like estrogen in preventing postmenopausal osteoporosis. A very interesting article by Dr. Stefano Palomba published in *Fertility and Sterility* described a study of seventy postmenopausal women with uterine fibroids. Many women with fibroids consider taking standard hormone replacement regimens (such as Premarin and Provera) after menopause but are concerned that HRT might increase the size of their fibroids. Since raloxifene helps to prevent osteoporosis, the investigators hoped that it would do this without increasing the size or symptoms of uterine fibroids. Happily enough, this was exactly what happened. Of thirty-one women who took 60 mg a day of raloxifene, 83 percent had a reduction in the size of their uterus and in their uterine fibroids after just over two years of treatment. Raloxifene did not cause thickening of the endometrium, an early sign of endometrial hyperplasia.

In our opinion, this limited study with raloxifene is one of the most promising studies of drug treatment for uterine fibroids. Unfortunately, these results were seen only in *postmenopausal* women; the drug has *not* been studied in premenopausal women. Raloxifene is an FDA-approved drug, and it has been used for many years to treat osteoporosis without evidence of ill effects on the *postmenopausal* women who take it. Because, as previously mentioned, any drug treatment for fibroids must be considered a long-term treatment, more and better data of raloxifene is needed before it can be routinely prescribed. We would not recommend taking raloxifene outside of the confines of a clinical trial aimed at investigating its effects on fibroids, but we're hopeful that a large trial like this will soon be underway.

Androgen Therapy

Danazol (Danocrine) is an older synthetic steroid that is chemically similar to testosterone and acts in a similar way to Lupron. Danazol reduces estrogen levels and stops ovulation and menstruation. While danazol reduces abnormally high levels of bleeding (and causes symptoms of menopause in many women who take it), it has not been demonstrated to shrink fibroids.

Gestrinone is an androgen-like steroid hormone believed to act against both estrogen and progesterone. Although not approved for use in the United States, it is used in Europe where at least three studies have tested it on women with uterine fibroids. The drug resulted in a decrease in fibroid size in about two-thirds of the women who took it. Of women with fibroids who also had heavy bleeding, about half stopped their bleeding over the course of several months of treatment. In one study, fibroids shrank an average of 40 percent after a year of treatment, and they did not immediately regrow. An estimated 89 percent of women maintained the decrease in uterine size for eighteen months. However, an alarming 40 to 93 percent of women reported masculinizing side effects including deepening voice, body hair growth, weight gain, and fluid retention. Gestrinone also caused acne in almost 50 percent of the patients who used it, although this effect seemed to decrease after one year of use. These side effects make it unlikely that gestrinone will be a useful treatment for fibroids.

Interferon

Laboratory studies show that interferon-alpha and interferon-beta have a potential beneficial effect on fibroids, although trials on humans have not been conducted for this purpose. In one recent case, a woman who was treated with interferon for hepatitis-C for seven months also saw shrinkage of a fibroid from 202 cubic centimeters to 29 cubic centimeters, and the fibroid became even smaller several months after therapy was complete. Interferon is frightfully expensive and carries significant risks from side effects. Development of this drug with specific application to fibroids along with appropriate clinical trials would need to be carried out before interferon could be considered a reasonable option for any woman with fibroids.

Investigational Medical Therapies

Therapy	Names	Risks	Benefits
Anti-progesterone	Mifeprix (mifepristone, RU-486)	Hyperplasia, mild menopausal symptoms.	Shrinks fibroids.
Selective estrogen receptor modulators (SERMs)	Raloxifene (Evista) Tamoxifen (Nolvadex)	May cause birth defects, endometrial cancer, or hyperplasia (Tamoxifen), or stimulate fibroid growth.	May shrink fibroids or prevent new ones from occurring.
Androgens	Danazol (Danocrine) Gestrinone	Menopausal symptoms and acne; masculinizing side effects including deepening voice, body hair growth, weight gain, and fluid retention.	Reduce estrogen levels and stop ovulation and menstruation thereby controlling abnormal bleeding.

Interferon	Interferon-alpha	Lengthy list of side	Shrinks fibroids.
	Interferon-beta	effects including flulike	
		symptoms, nausea,	
		severe depression,	
		thyroid disease,	
		gastrointestinal	
		problems, and	
		decreased white blood	
		cells and platelets.	

Chapter 11

❖

Uterine Fibroid Embolization

This chapter looks at the most promising new medical option for some women with fibroids—technically known as bilateral transcatheter uterine artery embolization, and more commonly known as uterine fibroid embolization, or UFE. Pioneered in the United States by our group, embolization is perhaps the safest of all emerging medical technologies if the symptoms of fibroids must be controlled by invasive means.

With UFE, a plastic tube called a catheter is threaded through a small opening in the skin into the femoral artery. The procedure is monitored with a type of X-ray machine called a fluoroscope; contrast dye is used to make the blood vessels visible. The tip of the catheter is guided to the point where the uterine arteries branch off from the arteries on each side of the uterus. Here, from 100 to 1,500 milligrams of small plastic particles are released into the bloodstream. If needed, from one to three gelatin sponge pledgets are also released. These particles move with the flow of blood, creating a miniature logjam in the arteries that eliminates the blood flow to fibroids, allowing them to shrink.

Embolization is a very effective treatment for bleeding, and it results in significant reductions in fibroid size. Although UFE does not physically remove fibroids, fibroids may not grow back to their previous size, as may happen with current drug treatments. Uterine fibroid embolization is performed by a medical specialist called an *interventional radiologist* (IR) who should be board eligible or certified by the American Board of Radiology. Recognized as a medical specialty in 1992, there are now more than four thousand interventional radiologists practicing in the United States, including many skilled at uterine fibroid embolization.

Are IRs Trained in Gynecology?

Most IRs have only limited gynecological training, which they received in medical school. Obstetrics and gynecology is usually a required rotation in medical school lasting several months. A few interventional radiologists have acquired additional training in gynecology following their radiology training and do perform gynecologic exams, although this is rare. Physicians usually make their decision about what specialty to go into in their third or fourth year of medical school and are required to apply for internship and residency in the fall of their fourth year.

Compared to hysterectomy or myomectomy, surgical procedures that have been performed for well over one hundred years in the United States, UFE is a relatively new procedure. Even so, uterine fibroid embolization has proven to be a safe, reputable procedure with a solid track record. More than ten thousand procedures have been performed to date in the United States, and the success rate has been quite high. Although not fully accepted quite yet, embolization could help many more women deal with fibroids; some insurance companies still don't cover it as a standard treatment. In our opinion, uterine fibroid embolization should *always* be presented as a treatment option for women with syptomatic fibroids who require therapy. Embolization is often the most attractive option for a woman who wishes to retain her uterus but in whom surgery might be difficult, such as a woman with a number of small fibroids buried in the uterine muscle that would be difficult for a surgeon to remove completely and safely. This is particularly true for women not strongly interested in future fertility. It is also an option for some women with larger fibroids who don't want surgery.

WHO CHOOSES THIS PROCEDURE?

A recent multicenter clinical trial in Ontario surveyed 555 women who chose uterine fibroid embolization, of whom 66 percent were white, 23 percent were black, and 11 percent were of other races. This group of women had an average age of forty-three; more than one-third were under forty. Approximately 85 percent were working outside the home, two-thirds were university educated, and more than half were married or with a regular partner. Before embolization, 80 percent of these women reported heavy menstrual bleeding, and 75 percent reported pelvic pain. Significant numbers reported other symptoms such as urinary complaints, pain during intercourse, a limited ability to exercise, and absence from work because of fibroids. Researchers in Canada concluded that large numbers of women suffering from the symptoms of fibroids are averse to surgery and actively seeking alternatives.

It is important to keep in mind that uterine fibroid embolization is a major medical procedure. All major medical procedures carry significant risks, including the risk of death. Risk of death with uterine fibroid embolization is currently approximated to be one in five thousand women compared to one in one thousand women who undergo hysterectomy. Most women experience side effects after the procedure, such as pain and nausea, with major complications happening much more rarely. Although the vast majority of women sail easily through this procedure, perhaps one in every ten women will have either a minor or a major complication.

The Society of Interventional Radiology (SIR), in partnership with the Cardiovascular and Interventional Radiology Research and Education Foundation (CIRREF), is currently funding one of the largest fibroid registry projects ever undertaken. This project will identify and assess UFE's range of complications, long-term durability, and impact on fertility and quality of life and collect information allowing researchers to compare UFE to other fibroid therapies. Interventional radiology practices all over the United States are enrolling their patients in the registry and collecting a great deal of information about the patients' histories, procedural data, postprocedural results, and complications.

Fibroid Registry for Outcomes Data (FIBROID) Research Questions

- Is UFE a safe treatment for leiomyomata? What is the incidence of minor and serious short-term complications?
- Is UFE an effective treatment for leiomyomata? What is the likelihood of symptom relief?
- How durable is the treatment? What is the likelihood of a subsequent procedure or medical therapy to treat recurrent symptoms of leiomyomata?
- What is the likelihood that a woman who undergoes UFE and plans subsequent pregnancy will be able to conceive and deliver a subsequent intrauterine pregnancy?
- Is there a difference in outcome based on device (product size, primary and secondary embolic material) used?

- Are there certain patient subgroups at higher risk or that have an increased likelihood of treatment benefits?
- What number of procedures should be recommended for training and to maintain skills?

Source: UFE FIBROID Registry, www.fibroidregistry.org.

Over two thousand patients have been enrolled in the registry, and the information collected thus far is currently being correlated. The goal of this project is to register and track both the short-term and long-term outcomes of women choosing UFE for their fibroids. The registry is expected to collect baseline and thirty-day follow-up information on approximately 2,500 women per year. Primary "core" sites involved in the study will possibly follow as many as nine hundred women for two to five years, depending on available funding. To date, there have been no significant surprises in the registry. In other words, previously reported safety and efficacy reports do seem to be holding up in this large study.

Society of Interventional Radiology (SIR)

The Society of Interventional Radiology (SIR), formerly known as the Society of Cardiovascular and Interventional Radiology (SCVIR), is dedicated to promoting the educational teaching missions of Interventional Radiology. It holds a major meeting once a year and multiple minor meetings per year. The primary focus of these meetings is to teach the interventional radiology community the latest technical skills and share medical research outcomes in all the different areas of this subspecialty of radiology.

Penny was twenty-eight years old when she was diagnosed with fibroids. During an annual exam, her gynecologist mentioned the presence of a benign tumor, told her that many women had them, and told her not

to worry about it. The doctor breezed out of the room, leaving Penny worried and puzzled. When told she had a benign tumor, Penny immediately feared cancer. "I was a twenty-eight-year-old who didn't know what benign meant. Besides, who wants a tumor growing in them?" she asked.

An experienced technical writer, Penny raced to the library and began researching fibroids. The medical books told her that fibroids weren't cancer. However, the most worrisome thing was that all the books indicated that hysterectomy would be the ultimate solution.

Time passed, and the fibroid grew. Penny had another child. This pregnancy was very uncomfortable, and the delivery was much more difficult and uncomfortable than her first had been because of the fibroid.

"Every checkup after that, I started getting recommendations to have a hysterectomy," Penny recalls. "I was still fairly young. I wanted more children. It distressed me that gynecologists told me I didn't need more children."

She asked all her doctors, "Can't the tumor just be removed?"

One after the other, they recommended hysterectomy.

Six years after being diagnosed with fibroids, a general practitioner gave thirty-four-year-old Penny her first ultrasound test establishing a baseline for her fibroids. The ultrasound showed four fibroids, the largest of which eventually grew to 12 centimeters. Her symptoms became severe. She suffered excessive menstrual bleeding. The fibroids triggered swelling in her legs and feet, and she suffered stress incontinence and back pain, all of which impacted her quality of life.

She just wanted to get the fibroids removed. At one point, Penny scheduled a myomectomy with a controversial female gynecologist in California, whose book she had read, but Penny canceled the surgery when she realized the doctor was being investigated by the state medical board.

"By this point, I was borderline suicidal. I had pretty much given up on life," Penny recalls. Her home life with her husband and children was extremely difficult. Her symptoms had more or less taken over her life. Her existence became a nightmare. Penny constantly took pain medication, yet saw no good way to end the pain.

Eventually, Penny learned about embolization and met with an interventional radiologist.

"The procedure was relatively simple. It went quickly. The whole thing lasted less than an hour, and most of that was spent watching them prepare the room," Penny recalls.

After the procedure, Penny experienced unusually strong cramping and pain. At one point, before she was adequately medicated, the pain was almost unbearable, but it passed. Overall, Penny's uterine fibroid embolization was successful, with the dominant fibroid shrinking almost in half—from 12 cm to about 7.5 cm. Every one of her symptoms from fibroids—bleeding, incontinence, back pain, and edema—was alleviated. Three years later Penny says she would still choose uterine fibroid embolization over hysterectomy.

Uterine fibroid embolization is minimally invasive compared to myomectomy or hysterectomy. It has an 85 percent clinical success rate, defined as a complete relief or substantial improvement of symptoms, with no additional operative procedures necessary. Although this is impressive, success rates could improve as physicians become more experienced with this new technique and treatment protocols are standardized.

Uterine fibroid embolization has several significant advantages over surgery. For one thing, it's quick. Fibroid embolizations have been done in as little as thirty minutes; in most women it takes between forty-five minutes and an hour and fifteen minutes to perform the procedure. Afterward, the women must lie down for about six hours. Hospital time averages one and a half days. Most women remain in the hospital only one day, and most return to work within a week. Total recovery time averages seven to fourteen days. Embolization is usually done under conscious sedation rather than under a general anesthetic, and as such carries less risk of a reaction to anesthesia. The incisions made in the body are a quarter inch or less, allowing for faster healing. Scarring is minimal.

Uterine fibroid embolization does not have a long history of use for fibroids, but midterm outcomes have been excellent, and it compares favorably with myomectomy. Many insurance companies are already covering it as a standard procedure, but a few still consider it experimental.

One woman we know already had one myomectomy, and when fibroids recurred, she wanted to avoid major surgery and try UFE. She went before the board of her HMO to ask them to allow her to have a uterine fibroid embolization. Trained as a nurse, she made a spectacular presentation to the appropriate committee at her insurance company, using visual aids and presenting plenty of facts. This woman had done her research, and she felt embolization was a safer and less invasive procedure for her. Although she made a good case for UFE, the insurance company board did not grant her request, and she was forced to choose between having a second myomectomy and having a hysterectomy.

Uterine fibroid embolization is not a highly invasive surgical procedure. However, in some ways, it may be compared to a myomectomy, which removes fibroids. While neither procedure removes the uterus, myomectomy removes fibroids while embolization only shrinks them by cutting off their blood supply. Unlike fibroid surgery, embolization rarely requires blood transfusions. Embolization may be safer than myomectomy, and it doesn't leave big scars on the skin or on the uterus. Treatment times and recovery times appear to be considerably shorter with embolization.

A 1998 study examined quality of life issues in a group of women who were treated for fibroids with symptoms of excessive bleeding and bulkiness. Three months after embolization, 79 percent of the women said they would definitely choose the procedure again, 15 percent would consider it, and 6 percent said they would choose another treatment. In this study, 88 percent of the women reported marked improvement in the symptom of abnormal bleeding, and 94 percent reported marked improvement in bulk symptoms.

How Does a Physician Train to Become an Interventional Radiologist?

The interventional radiologist typically will do a one-year internship in either medicine or surgery, or complete a transitional year in which multiple specialties are studied. The IR will then do a four-year diagnostic radiology residency followed by a one- to two-year fellowship. At the end of this training, the typical interventional radiologist will have performed five hundred to one thousand cases. (These numbers represent a broad array of treatments, however, and not just uterine fibroid embolization.) For fellowships, there is a specific criterion as to the total number of cases and the total number of specific types of cases that are performed.

In addition, three small studies have been conducted on women's sexual function after uterine fibroid embolization. All three studies concluded that the majority of women had improved sexual function or no change in sexuality at all. However, a small percentage—less than 10 percent—of women reported decreased intensity of orgasm following the procedure. Studies after hysterectomy have shown a similar percentage of women with decreased sexual function.

There are limitations and risks to uterine fibroid embolization, however, and not all women with fibroids are good candidates for this procedure. For instance, it is not currently recommended as first-line treatment for women who wish to conceive a child.

HOW IT WORKS

Uterine embolization shrinks fibroids without removing the uterus. This is possible because fibroids are almost exclusively supplied with blood and nutrients from the uterine arteries, which increase in size as fibroids grow. These arteries are "end arteries," like the arteries going into the kidneys, which is crucial for the success of the procedure ("end arteries" do not have significant collaterals—when they are blocked, blood cannot get around the blockade). The uterus itself has other sources of blood besides the uterine arteries, such as the ovarian arteries and other, smaller blood vessels. This makes it possible to cut off most of the fibroids' blood supply via the uterine arteries while leaving the uterus unharmed, since the normal uterus has a more extensive blood supply than the fibroids. This loss of blood supply (and nutrients) shrinks fibroids without cutting them out of the uterus, and the resulting shrinkage helps control bleeding and other symptoms.

Since this procedure takes place entirely inside of blood vessels, it may seem difficult to comprehend how an interventional radiologist even accomplishes the procedure. However, an interventional radiologist can navigate a catheter into an artery by watching the catheter within the artery under the fluoroscope. Although the artery is invisible, it can be visualized intermittently by injecting X-ray dye called *contrast* into the artery. There are also computer techniques that project an image of the artery onto the screen and overlay an image of the catheter, and the wire within the catheter onto the image of the artery. This technique is called *road mapping*, and it requires that the patient remain still.

The catheter is controlled from outside the body and usually has some sort of shape at the end such as a short hook. The catheter can be twisted on the outside thereby steering the tip of the catheter. Typically, the wire is advanced through the inside of the catheter out into the artery, and the catheter is then advanced over the wire. The wire is also steerable allowing the interventional radiologist to twist the wire on the outside of the body thereby directing the tip on the inside of the body.

Certificate of Added Qualification (CAQ)

The American Board of Radiology offers board certification in diagnostic radiology and also what is called a Certificate of Added Qualification in vascular and interventional radiology. A physician who holds this added board certification had substantial training and/or experience in interventional radiology and has passed a case file review and an oral board examination. This does not mean that a physician who does not have the certificate is unqualified, but it does indicate a certain level of advanced experience and knowledge in a person holding this certificate.

Variations in the Uterine Artery

For an experienced interventional radiologist, particularly one who has had experience in embolization procedures, uterine fibroid embolization is not generally a difficult procedure. However, some women do have particularly tortuous (curvy) uterine arteries, which makes catheterization difficult. For some of these women the procedure can stretch from the typical forty-five minutes to one hour out to several hours. A variety of different techniques using microcatheters and microwires need to be applied to accomplish catheterization of this type of artery.

> Karen, a woman in her forties, agreed to undergo uterine fibroid embolization with several physician observers present. Of course, the physician observers had been told that the procedure time was usually around fifty minutes and that there had never been a technical failure in our practice. As it turned out, the patient had an extremely tortuous uterine artery on one side with a very unfavorable angle at the origin. Despite a procedure time that lasted between two and three hours and the use of multiple microcatheters and microwires and various other angiography tricks, catheterizing the uterine artery on one side was never accomplished (although one side was catheterized successfully). Surprisingly, in short-term follow-up the patient had a significant improvement in symptoms.

> This was probably because the uterus had a markedly uneven blood supply and the artery that was not embolized was the smaller of the two. On angiography, it looked as though the predominant blood supply was from the side that was successfully embolized.

Anatomic abnormalities of the uterine artery are unusual. However, variants do exist that can create a "shared" blood flow between what would usually be completely separate blood vessels. This condition is called arterial anastomosis. The uterine artery usually originates as a major branch of the anterior trunk of the internal iliac artery. Rarely, a single uterine artery, and even more rarely both uterine arteries, will essentially be replaced by branches coming from the ovarian arteries. In addition, quite rarely, there may be more than one uterine artery on a side.

Anastomosis between the ovarian and uterine arteries is of considerable concern, as embolic material may flow to the ovaries during the time of UFE and potentially damage healthy, functional ovaries. Unfortunately, at this time there is no widely available and accepted method to determine the degree of arterial anastomosis between the ovarian and uterine arteries prior to embolization. Some groups are working diligently on developing MRI/MRA (magnetic resonance imaging and angiography) in order to help identify these connections.

It is now well known that the embolization of only one uterine artery increases the chance of failure. It does not mean that the patient will definitely fail therapy—many patients have had only a single uterine artery embolized and have had a successful outcome when the principal supply to the fibroids was from the artery embolized. Nevertheless, it is important to embolize both arteries if possible. Sometimes it can be very technically difficult to catheterize one of the arteries. In time, however, this artery will enlarge and the patient can be brought back in a few weeks for embolization.

Like some of the other physician groups experienced in UFE, we have seen only one patient who had a missing uterine artery. We have also had one patient with two uterine arteries on the left side, which was quite a surprise. Approximately 1 percent of patients have significant and obvious connections between the uterine artery and the ovarian artery visualized on uterine arteriography. However, more than one half of patients have a communication between the ovarian and uterine arteries that is not visualized on angiography. In some cases, the fundus, or top of the uterus, has been largely supplied by the ovarian arteries. The Stanford group has shown that approximately 10 percent of patients will have some blood supply to the uterus from the ovarian arteries. Occasionally, the sheer size of the uterine artery—as well as the fibroids—is sincerely surprising.

Variations in Technique

When we started the embolization program at the UCLA Medical Center, we embolized to completion. This meant that the uterine artery was filled with embolization material until there was no remaining flow within the artery. This was consistent with what the French had done originally and with how most other arteries are embolized. There was some concern that if the artery was not completely embolized, this would increase the likelihood of leaving blood flowing to the fibroids, thereby not resulting in their death.

Some interventional radiologists embolize only partially.

This means that they fill the uterine artery until they don't see blood flow in what is called the ascending uterine artery or in the branches off the ascending uterine artery, but they allow some remaining blood flow at the base of the uterus in what is called the lower uterine segment. So far, studies have suggested that these two techniques do not differ in terms of efficacy or safety, but there is no proof that this is true. Proof would require a direct prospective randomized comparison of the two techniques.

Embolic Particles

Three types of particles are used to embolize uterine fibroids: polyvinyl alcohol foam (PVA), Gelfoam, and Embospheres.

The most common embolic material, PVA, has been used for several decades in a wide variety of innovative radiological procedures involving almost every part of the body. PVA is available in the United States from four different manufacturers under a variety of trade names. The material has been used throughout the body to stop bleeding and to stop tumors from further growth. It has a long record of safety without any substantive evidence that it causes allergic or other problems and appears to be completely safe, with no adverse effects on the body.

Gelfoam, which is a trade name for gelatin sponge, is a material that has also been around for quite a long time and used to stop excessive bleeding during surgery. In interventional radiology embolization procedures, Gelfoam is cut into small pieces and then injected directly into a blood vessel to encourage blood clotting and to block off the blood vessel. This material is frequently used to stop bleeding that occurs from fractured bones in the pelvis. It has also long been used to stop bleeding after childbirth or after gynecologic surgery or because of an abnormal placenta. Gelfoam is thought to be a temporary material that the body reabsorbs within a couple of weeks, which is usually associated with reopening of the blocked artery.

Embospheres is the trade name for the calibrated microspheres or trisacryl gelatin microspheres manufactured by Biosphere. This particle has been approved for use in Europe for nearly a decade. It is currently also available in the United States and has been used in hundreds of patients with fibroids. Embospheres are easier to inject and less likely to clog up the catheter than PVA is. They also result in a more predictable level of occlusion, or cutting off the blood supply to the fibroids. At this time, Embospheres generally appear to be safe. However, a substance in Embospheres contains a gold compound to make the particles easier to visualize on angiography. This substance may be associated with increased allergic reactions, but more research is necessary to absolutely associate the reported side effects with this substance.

Although at least one health organization has suggested that these embolic particles may cause cancer, there is absolutely no evidence in the research or published medical literature to suggest that PVA foam particles, Gelfoam, or Embospheres are carcinogenic. All of these materials have undergone extensive evaluations, both in animal models and in humans, and have *not* been shown to cause cancer.

DISTINGUISHED HISTORY

Embolization as a medical procedure first came into wide use in the 1960s and 1970s as a treatment for excessive bleeding from operations, childbirth, or tumors. It is now an accepted technique for treating those conditions. Its effects on fibroids were discovered by a fortunate accident in France about ten years ago. At that time, Dr. Jacques Ravina, Dr. Jean Merland, and their colleagues observed that patients with fibroids who were treated for bleeding before surgery with uterine artery embolization also experienced shrinkage of fibroids and relief from their symptoms. These women began to call Dr. Ravina to cancel their fibroid surgeries. He put two and two together. This was an insight of epic proportions for women with fibroids.

The first formal study of this new technique was conducted in Europe and published in the prestigious British medical journal the *Lancet* in 1995. In Dr. Ravina's first report, eleven of sixteen Parisian women who underwent embolization reported complete resolution of their symptoms. Another three of the sixteen had partial improvement. Two women had no improvement and ultimately required surgery. These were surprisingly good results. After the procedure, the Parisian women reported no complications other than pelvic pain. Time in the hospital was never more than thirty-six hours. Ultrasound assessment after the procedure confirmed that the women experienced between a 20 and 80 percent reduction in fibroid size after three months. A subsequent larger study, also conducted in France, found that 89 percent of women with excessive bleeding reverted to a normal menstrual cycle following embolization.

As word of the impressive French successes spread around the world, several U.S. medical centers, including those at the University of California at Los Angeles Medical Center, Roxborough Community Hospital, and Georgetown University, and several hospitals in Canada, began investigating this exciting new technique. At the UCLA Medical Center, investigation into uterine fibroid embolization was begun in 1996, with very encouraging early results that were in line with published reports from France.

UAE OR UFE?

UAE stands for uterine artery embolization and means exactly what it says: the introduction of material designed to block off the uterine artery. This is the technically correct term for the procedure that women undergo for the treatment of uterine fibroids.

Uterine fibroid embolization, or UFE, is a term that arose to help women understand what exactly was being treated. It is true that during a uterine artery embolization, the fibroids are embolized. But it is also true that the entire uterus is embolized. This begs the question of why the uterus doesn't have more problems following the embolization than fibroids do. As discussed earlier, fibroid arteries are essentially end arteries, such as those that occur in the kidneys. This means that no significant connection exists between fibroid arteries and other arteries, which are collateral arteries. Therefore, when these arteries are blocked off, fibroids have no significant blood supply and subsequently die. This is unlike the normal myometrial tissue of the uterus, where there is significant collateral flow from one part of the uterus to the other. In other words, blood flow can get around the embolization in the normal tissue but not in the fibroids.

RESULTS

At the UCLA Medical Center, eight of our first nine patients to undergo UFE experienced improvement, including three women with *complete* resolution of all symptoms. Reductions of fibroid size averaged 40 percent. Reductions in the size of the largest fibroids averaged 65 percent, with results convincingly demonstrated on ultrasound.

In subsequent research, uterine fibroid embolization was employed on a larger group of fifty-nine women, fifty-six of whom suffered from excessive bleeding and forty-seven of whom had pain before the procedure. After embolization, a startling 81 percent had improvements in their symptoms. In addition, 92 percent of these women had reductions in the size of their uterus and in the volume of their largest fibroids, averaging between 42 and 50 percent. However, it was necessary to repeat the procedure in two of the fifty-nine women, one of whom had a successful outcome while the other did not. As in France, all women experienced some pelvic pain after the procedure, varying from the pain of menstrual cramps to the pain of childbirth. All received medication to help them control the pain. Four women expelled submucosal fibroids from their vaginas. Moreover, even though the presence of adenomyosis (see chapter 3) was believed to doom the procedure to failure, we found to our surprise that three women with adenomyosis had a successful outcome in our trials, although three others did not.

In the Georgetown University studies published in 1999, fifty women who underwent embolization for fibroids experienced an average of 48 percent decreased uterine volume, and a 78 percent reduction in largest fibroid volume as confirmed by magnetic resonance imaging. Menstrual bleeding problems improved in 89 percent of patients, and pelvic pain and pressure improved in 96 percent of patients.

Because of this research, we can confidently state that between 81 and 94 percent of women who undergo uterine fibroid embolization experience improvement or resolution of primary fibroid-related symptoms. Bleeding is controlled in 86 to 90 percent of women, and reductions in uterine size and fibroid volume range from 40 to 61 percent. These results compare favorably with myomectomy, but women who undergo embolization have less scarring and shorter hospitalization and recovery times.

LARGE FIBROIDS

For women with particularly large fibroids—that is, with a uterine size greater than a twenty-week pregnancy—the current medical thinking is that myomectomy is a better choice than embolization. However, many women with extremely large fibroids have also had successful uterine fibroid embolizations.

We remember one patient with a very large nine-liter uterus and serious symptoms. As a point of reference, a liter is about the size of a quart of milk. After embolization the woman's uterus shrank to less than one and a half liters in size—a great reduction that made the patient ecstatic since she also experienced a significant reduction in her symptoms and a vastly improved quality of life.

Several other interventional radiologists have also reported success in treating women with larger fibroids, although the procedure is usually more successful in women with numerous smaller fibroids.

A few women with special situations have also undergone both uterine fibroid embolization and myomectomy. For women who have a substantial risk of bleeding, or women with a religious belief against using their own blood, such as Jehovah's Witnesses, a uterine fibroid embolization prior to myomectomy surgery to remove fibroids significantly reduces bleeding from fibroids and shrinks them. This double procedure allows these women to get through myomectomies without undergoing blood transfusions.

Deep Venous Thrombosis (DVT)

Women with abnormal bleeding and extremely large fibroids need to be particularly aware of a condition called deep venous (vein) thrombosis, or DVT. DVT refers to the formation of a thrombus (blood clot) within a deep vein, commonly in the thigh or calf but also the pelvis. This can have two serious consequences:

1. If the thrombus partially or completely blocks the flow of blood through the vein, blood begins to pool and build up below the site. Chronic swelling and pain may develop.

2. If the thrombus breaks free and travels through the veins, it can reach the lungs, where it is called a pulmonary embolism (PE). A pulmonary embolism is a potentially fatal condition that can kill within minutes to hours.

Women with large fibroids may have an increased deep venous thrombosis risk if they are inactive because of the compressive potential from the size of their fibroids or because of severe hemorrhage resulting in a depletion of blood vessel volume and stagnant blood flow through the veins. Patients like this should go immediately to the emergency room if they notice that one or both of their legs are swollen and/or painful. Also, if they experience the acute onset of shortness of breath or sudden chest pain, particularly in the setting of a swollen leg, they should go immediately to the emergency room because they may have suffered a pulmonary embolism. Conditions that can lead to DVT include the following:

- Inactivity (from a sedentary job); a long trip, especially in a cramped space (e.g., economy class section of a plane); prolonged bed rest

- Heart failure or heart attack

- Being overweight, in poor physical condition, or older

- Trauma to an arm or leg (a fall) or injury to the vein (from injections or IV needles)

- Some cancers

- Varicose veins, pregnancy, abnormal uterine bleeding and/or large fibroids, or estrogen therapy

Preventing DVT

- Avoid sitting or standing for long periods without moving around.
- Inform your doctor if you have a history of varicose veins or DVT and take estrogen.
- Avoid tobacco.
- On trips, drink lots of fluids (no alcohol) and move about at least every hour. Exercise the legs in place if options for walking about are not available.
- If you are confined to a bed or a chair or work at a desk job, stretch often.

Source: National Uterine Fibroids Foundation.

We are aware of at least one patient who died after developing DVT and a pulmonary embolism while awaiting treatment for her fibroids. In addition, although the precise underlying reasons are unclear, two patients (out of the entire number of UFEs performed in the world to date) have died following fibroid embolization due to pulmonary embolism, when a clot traveled from a vein into the lungs some time after the procedure.

RISKS OF THE PROCEDURE

Uterine fibroid embolization is generally safe, but there are risks and side effects from any invasive procedure. Mortality is the greatest risk, but statistically speaking, embolization is safer than hysterectomy, which is in itself considered quite a safe operation. In the world literature, only two deaths have been reported from embolization, which is remarkably low considering this is a new technique. We now calculate mortality at one in every five thousand procedures, which is the lowest risk of any invasive technique. For hysterectomy, the risk is approximately one in one thousand.

Contraindications for UFE

If you have any of the following conditions, you should definitely *not* undergo uterine fibroid embolization:

- Active endometriosis

- Significant former therapeutic pelvic radiation
- Various vascular diseases (check with the interventional radiologist for more details)
- Pelvic infection

Additional issues of concern that should be discussed thoroughly prior to choosing UFE are as follows:

- Irreversible coagulation disorders
- Severe kidney problems
- Severe contrast dye allergy
- Desire for future fertility

In approximately 5 percent of cases, however, women have gone into a premature menopause or ovarian failure after embolization due to *nontarget embolization*. This may be the result of embolic material flowing into the ovaries through connections between the uterine and ovarian arteries. These connections are difficult to visualize angiographically in most women. The effect seems to be age dependent, with the ovaries being compromised due to UFE in less than 1 percent of patients under thirty-five years of age but possibly greater than 33 percent of patients over the age of forty-eight.

Pain

Patient pain history, pain expectations, and medication history are extremely relevant to a patient's experience of pain following a procedure. For example, a patient who has been on narcotics long term (for whatever reason) will have a significant narcotic tolerance, and therefore the amount of narcotics necessary following UFE (or any surgical procedure) will be much greater. If a patient has a high expectation of having pain following procedure, this may increase the likelihood she reports pain following the procedure and may also increase her need for pain medication. In addition, patients who have had chronic pain lasting longer than three months experience pain differently than do those who have not.

Pelvic pain after the procedure is the most common side effect, along with nausea, although both are transitory. Some pain can be expected, so we recommend that women remain in the hospital overnight. It should be noted that some practitioners perform UFE on an outpatient basis. Pain may be minimized by the use of mild anti-inflammatory drugs such as ibuprofen before and after the procedure. Intravenous narcotics are used during the procedure, and patient-controlled analgesia (PCA) pumps are used afterward for patients who need stronger drugs for pain control. So far, all pelvic pain after the procedure has completely resolved in most patients within two weeks. Most are pain free within a week. About a third of patients develop a fever of 100.4°F or higher. Among the women who develop fever, about 15 percent develop a significant "postembolization syndrome" consisting of fever and high white blood cell count, which can be managed by medical treatment.

Sloughing of a submucosal fibroid has occurred in about 5 percent of patients. This is generally noticed first in the form of sudden cramplike pain and possibly a foul-smelling vaginal discharge. In most cases, the dying (necrotic) fibroid material passes harmlessly within forty-eight hours. If the fibroid the uterus is attempting to pass becomes lodged in the cervix and becomes infected, it can be removed by the physician with a D&C. If an infected fibroid is not removed in a timely manner, however, a hysterectomy is necessary. In Dr. Ravina's early studies, one patient developed this complication. In a later study of fifty-three women who underwent embolization, one woman experienced this complication. As a result, we now recommend that submucosal fibroids growing on a narrow stalk be removed surgically before embolization. Generally, this is accomplished through hysteroscopic myomectomy, a procedure discussed in chapter 12.

The amount of radiation in an average uterine fibroid embolization is 20 rads—about ten times the radiation received during a pelvic CAT scan. This is almost never enough radiation to affect fertility or significantly increase the risk of cancer. The only complication involving radiation we have seen is one woman whose embolization took more than four hours; she developed second- to third-degree burns as a result of her exposure to radiation. Since radiation has a cumulative effect, it should be minimized as much as possible by the interventional radiologist.

Approximately 5 percent of patients have a small amount of bleeding or a minor bruise on the groin after the procedure. Rarely, more serious vascular damage is possible from the angiographic technique. An infection in the groin, or kidney failure due to the use of the contrast dye, are possibilities, although serious complications of this type are quite rare.

We know of one woman who achieved relief from fibroids through embolization, but suffered a regrowth of the fibroids after beginning hormone replacement therapy. It is not known if this will be a typical experience or not.

Rare but serious complications from embolization include uterine infection, uterine perforation, uterine rupture during labor, uterine death, arterial injury, damage to other pelvic organs other than the ovaries, sexual dysfunction, major allergic reaction, and death. Pelvic infections that do not respond to antibiotics and require a subsequent hysterectomy have occurred in one-half of 1 percent of patients.

Embolization

Benefits	Risks
Does not remove uterus	Complications may occur
Shrinks fibroids/alleviates pressure symptoms and urinary incontinence	Does not remove fibroids
Controls bleeding	Radiation exposure
Less time in hospital	Potential for induced menopause/ ovarian failure
Minimal recovery time	Transitory pelvic pain

REALISTIC OUTCOME EXPECTATIONS

The main outcome expectation following uterine fibroid embolization is that bleeding, pain, or bulk symptoms such as pressure on the bladder and rectum are significantly improved. These improvements may occur even if the fibroids do not shrink substantially. Although the average fibroid volume reduction is approximately 50 percent, many patients, particularly those with larger fibroids, may not achieve this reduction, although they do have substantial improvement in their symptoms.

Even if the fibroid does not shrink substantially, it usually changes in consistency from a very hard mass to something very soft and more Jell-O–like. This can result in a marked decrease in the feeling of having a mass inside the pelvis and may result in decreased bulk symptoms including a swollen abdomen. However, if you have large fibroids and a "flat tummy" is what you want, then a myomectomy (removal of the fibroid tumors) or a hysterectomy may be a better treatment choice.

FERTILITY

An uncommon but significant side effect to UFE is early menopause or complete ovarian failure, which eliminates the possibility of having more children. This has occurred in approximately 5 percent of all women in research studies, when arteries feeding the ovaries were blocked by nontarget embolization. For this reason, we do not generally recommend embolization for women who seek to have children. However, we also know of several women who have become pregnant after embolization. We recommend embolization to women who desire children only in the following three cases:

1. When previous myomectomy and hormonal therapies have failed, and hysterectomy has been recommended to address significant problems related to fibroids.
2. When the size or placement of fibroids is such that a myomectomy would most likely not be successful or likely result in hysterectomy because of probable complications.
3. The patient is fully aware of the risks and benefits of all alternatives and refuses surgery.

Two small studies have shown that women who have undergone Gelfoam embolization for postpartum bleeding have suffered no ill effects on fertility. However, this is a different form of embolization, and results may not apply to other techniques. No long-term studies have been done with uterine fibroid embolization, which uses more permanent materials.

The issue of fertility needs further study before embolization can be recommended for women who want to have children.

LEIOMYOSARCOMA

One concern some women have about fibroid embolization is the possibility that a tumor believed to be a fibroid is actually a cancerous tumor, such as a leiomyosarcoma. Instead of embolizing a fibroid, what if the uterine tumor is actually a leiomyosarcoma? Leiomyosarcoma is a malignant and often fatal disease. Fortunately, it is quite rare, occurring in approximately one in a thousand patients seen for fibroids. However, it is age dependent, and the chance of having it does rise as an individual grows older.

At this time, no reliable way exists to distinguish a fibroid from a leiomyosarcoma. If a patient actually has a leiomyosarcoma, it will typically continue to grow after the embolization procedure. Because of continued growth and symptoms, this usually will lead to a hysterectomy. Sadly, whether the patient has the hysterectomy instead of the embolization or has the hysterectomy a few months after embolization does not usually change the ultimate outcome. Uterine leiomyosarcoma is an aggressive cancer. It typically spreads to other parts of the body and is relatively nonresponsive to all treatments currently available.

Questions to Ask Your Interventional Radiologist

- Are you board eligible or certified in interventional radiology?
- How many uterine fibroid embolizations have you performed?
- What are the results of your fibroid embolizations so far, and how often have complications occurred?
- How effective is UFE in shrinking the types of fibroids I have?
- What steps will you take to minimize my exposure to radiation?
- What medications will be used to treat pain, both in the hospital and once released?
- How long should I expect to be released from work to recover from UFE?

- What kind of follow-up care is typical, and who should I return to or consult with after the procedure for additional care, my gynecologist or you?
- Can you provide the names and phone numbers of former patients who might be willing to talk to me about this procedure?

PREOPERATIVE PREPARATION FOR UFE

A little preparation goes a long way. The night before your procedure, eat sensibly, something easy to digest. Something light makes sense, such as a romaine salad, as it has plenty of iron and fiber. Because of pain medications prescribed with this procedure, bowel activity may be slow afterward. Eating a high-fiber meal prior to the procedure may be important and is certainly a positive step you can take to help your body out in this regard. *Do not eat or drink anything past midnight.* Although the anesthetic used is local, it is still important to follow this rule.

One day before the procedure, prepare your bedside with the following:

- Clean sheets
- Tissues
- Fresh nightgown and slippers
- Heating pad
- Thermometer
- Phone and all emergency phone contact information
- Postoperative instructions
- Light reading

Inpatient vs. Outpatient UFE

When we first started our UFE program at the UCLA Medical Center, we decided to perform embolization on an outpatient basis. Soon, we discovered that a very high percentage of our patients were calling back in the middle of the night, usually with problems associated with pain. We then moved our practice toward admitting all patients overnight—with some patients staying two nights. Occasionally, a patient will stay even longer than two nights. Many other fibroid embolization practices have also adopted the policy of admitting patients. However, recently, several practices have begun doing UFE on an outpatient basis. This has met with some success, probably because of the improved pain management strategies now being used by physicians performing UFE.

Prepare your kitchen for when you come home:

- Limit dairy products (may cause constipation)
- Prune juice and raisins
- Metamucil (gentle fiber product to help with constipation)
- Tea bags
- Light, healthy foods (sliced turkey, bread, soups/broths, salads)
- Crushed ice

Prepare your car for the ride home after the procedure:

- Pillows (You may want to lie down in the back of your vehicle, and several pillows for support could ease your comfort.)
- Plastic bag (in case of nausea on the ride home)
- Comfortable, loose clothes and slip-on shoes

Generally, you may be kept in bed for six to eight hours after the procedure. This prevents you from moving the leg or attempting to walk around, giving the catheter insertion site time to clot off.

At the hospital:

- Ask a family member or partner to obtain and fill your prescription for pain relief when you're dropped off for the procedure so that you do not have to stop on the way home.

- Prepare a copy of important phone numbers and store them in a convenient place during the procedure. Be sure to find out who to call and for what, specifically, in terms of the procedure and recovery period.
- If your doctor is unavailable following the procedure, ask for the name and number of an alternative physician to call and add it to your phone list.
- Clarify all matters related to the procedure (including key contact information needed for your phone list) the morning prior to your UFE.

At home after the procedure:

- Take all pain relievers prescribed for you.
- Use heating pads. Place one over your abdomen and another under it, if necessary. Do not sleep with a heating pad in direct contact with the skin because burns may result.
- Limit your movement; take it slow, and save all household activity for another time. Limit your bending if possible.
- Avoid heavy lifting.
- Seek assistance and move slowly when trying to get up into a seated position.
- Eat. You may not want to, but your body needs nutrients to heal. Continue taking vitamins and iron supplements as well.
- Avoid alcohol (particularly while taking any prescribed medications), aspirin, and any foods that might "bind" your bowels (e.g., dairy products).

- Take the time necessary to simply heal and take care of yourself.

During the week following your procedure, watch for the following and report any or all of these signs to your physician, should they occur:

- Temperatures over 100.6°F (check it two or three times a day)
- Dizziness
- Swelling
- Bleeding at the catheter insertion site
- Return of fever or pain *after* symptoms have subsided (possibly weeks to months after the procedure)

If you happen to experience the very rare occurrence of bleeding at the catheter insertion site, you can generally stop the bleeding by pressing one finger on the site and two fingers upstream, above the puncture site. If bleeding continues, seek assistance and head to the emergency room for additional care.

Can an IR Manage Fibroid Patients Alone, Without a Gynecologist?

Patients with significant symptoms due to or in addition to their fibroids require a thorough gynecologic history and physical. Interventional radiologists do not usually have the appropriate training to perform a good gynecologic examination unless they have done a prior OB/GYN residency or taken additional postgraduate training. In addition, patients require ongoing OB/GYN history and physicals following the embolization procedure. The typical IR is not usually qualified to provide this service. Finally, some patients may experience symptoms such as a passing fibroid getting stuck at the cervix, which may require gynecologic intervention such as D&C and/or hysteroscopy performed by a technically skilled gynecologist.

AFTER EMBOLIZATION

We recommend good, basic follow-up medical treatment after embolization. This includes follow-up visits with your physician at one week (by telephone is okay), six weeks, six months, and a year after the procedure. To track the effects of the procedure on fibroids, we also recommend that you have ultrasound or MRI exams at six months, a year, and annually (if indicated) thereafter even though fibroids usually remain under control.

Embolization vs. Surgery

The following comparisons may be made from existing research studies, relating the two most common surgeries for fibroids, hysterectomy and myomectomy, to uterine fibroid embolization.

Symptom	UFE	Myomectomy	Hysterectomy
Menorrhagia (% of women seeing improvement)	90%	81%	100%
Transfusion necessary	<1%	10–32%	2–13%
Hospitalization (average # of days)	1.5	3.3	4.2 (abdominal) 2.8 (vaginal)
Recovery time	7–14 days	6 weeks (abdominal)	6 weeks

Uterine fibroid embolization is a legitimate choice for women who cannot control their symptoms with lifestyle changes or midlevel therapies such as prescription drugs. Uterine fibroid embolization has a high level of success at controlling symptoms and reducing uterine bulkiness. Compared with other invasive procedures, embolization is safer and less invasive than hysterectomy, and comparable to myomectomy in many ways. For many women, uterine fibroid embolization may be the superior choice. We need further study to determine exactly which women would benefit most from uterine fibroid embolization and which should be steered toward other options. Another option for many women, myomectomy—a surgery that removes fibroids—is the topic of the next chapter.

Chapter 12

Myomectomy

Myomectomy is a surgical technique that removes fibroids and leaves the uterus intact. Although much less frequently recommended and performed than hysterectomy, myomectomy has a number of advantages over removing the uterus, as well as some drawbacks. Most myomectomies are performed through a horizontal incision in the lower abdomen (a "bikini" cut). However, new procedures using miniature surgical instruments and high-tech tools such as lasers have made possible new forms of myomectomy that are less invasive.

Myomectomy and hysterectomy are two standard treatment options for women whose symptoms cannot be controlled with less invasive methods. Both surgeries are invasive procedures, and so are riskier than treatment with medications. Myomectomy removes fibroids but leaves the uterus intact. Hysterectomy, discussed in the next chapter, removes the uterus along with the fibroids. The pros and cons of each surgery should be carefully weighed and understood before you agree to either, since effects are permanent. Either treatment can be a good choice if symptoms from fibroids don't respond to medication or if using medications is not an option.

In other words, if your pain is not better, even with pain relievers, or you can't tolerate the side effects of medications, or your main problem is the *size* of the fibroids, then either treatment may provide relief from these problems. Myomectomy is the best choice for many women who want to save their uterus, or who wish to keep open the possibility of having children.

A forty-one-year-old woman named Judy first discovered she had fibroids five years ago. She went for a routine Pap smear and was startled when her doctor mentioned fibroids. Other women in her family had problems with fibroids. Her mother had them, but they were not treated. Her older sister had fibroids that were surgically removed. And here she was, with fibroids of her own.

"What should I do?" Judy asked her doctor.

"As long as you're not having symptoms, don't do anything," her doctor replied.

Three years later, after having one extremely heavy period, Judy was checked again by a new doctor, a young woman who had just begun her medical practice.

"Should I do something about these fibroids?" Judy asked.

An ultrasound examination revealed that the fibroids were pushing on one of her ureters, the tube that drains urine from the bladder to the kidney. When Judy asked about it, her doctor told her that her options were to live with it or get a myomectomy.

By this time, Judy was urinating a lot more than normal and suffering from heavy bleeding, especially during the first two days of her menstrual period. "I couldn't go through the night without getting up," Judy recalls. "I was feeling a great deal of pressure, like I was full all the time. The fibroids were extremely hard, and my stomach muscles felt tight all the time," she says.

Judy's father, a retired doctor, suggested that she have a urine analysis to check her kidney function. This test was normal. However, six months later, another ultrasound showed that Judy's uterus had grown to the size of a five-month pregnancy. She was referred to a young doctor at the university medical center. "As soon as I met him, I knew I was in the right hands," she recalls.

The new doctor explained her options and answered her questions, giving her information and time to choose a treatment. He explained to Judy that her fibroids were unfortunately too big for a laparoscopic myomectomy. Judy chose an abdominal myomectomy since she wanted to have children in the future.

Judy was put on GnRH agonist drugs for six months to help control her bleeding and shrink her fibroids, and eventually had surgery to remove the fibroids. "The last thing I said to my doctor was to please not take my uterus out," she recalls. The surgery went well, removing her fibroids without removing her uterus.

"I didn't want to get a hysterectomy," Judy says. "I like having my monthly periods and feeling like a young woman. I don't have any children now, but I'd kind of like to keep that window open. It was the best choice for me."

LIFE-SAVING SURGERY

In a limited number of cases, surgery for fibroids may save your life. Otherwise, it is elective or optional and designed to improve, rather than lengthen, life. In the following three cases, surgery will probably lengthen your life:

1. *Uncontrollable bleeding* is life threatening. Severe anemia leads to chronic exhaustion, dizziness, lowered resistance to disease, and increased risk of heart attack or heart failure. It is possible to bleed to death from fibroids. If massive bleeding can't be stopped by other means, invasive therapy is crucial. Depending on the circumstances, either a myomectomy, a hysterectomy, or an embolization might be recommended. If uncontrollable bleeding occurs during a myomectomy, hysterectomy and sometimes embolization are life-saving options.

2. *If the flow of urine out of the kidneys is blocked* by fibroids, dangerous pressure builds in the kidneys and may permanently injure them. This condition is extremely rare, but it can be treated with either a myomectomy, a hysterectomy, or an embolization. Tests to look for this rare problem include ultrasound, intravenous pyelogram (also called IVP) and MRI. Urine tests can check kidney function. If kidneys are functioning well despite the pressure, surgery is optional.

3. *The presence of cancer* is a third reason for surgery. Most types of uterine cancer require a hysterectomy. As explained in chapter 2, cancer involving uterine tumors (leiomyosarcoma) is very rare, affecting about one out of every thousand women with uterine tumors. However, this cancer does require a hysterectomy to treat it.

In most other situations, myomectomy is an elective procedure, a procedure you *choose* to undergo but which is not *required* to save your life. In these cases, while surgery may not save your life, it can improve your *quality* of life. For example, if symptoms are creating unbearable problems and interfering with your daily life, career, family life, or sexual activity so that it is not possible to enjoy life to the greatest extent possible, then you need some treatment. If less invasive therapies fail, uterine fibroid embolization, myomectomy, or hysterectomy are all very likely to make your life better.

If you want to have more children, and fibroids are keeping you from getting pregnant, the best choice is likely to be myomectomy since uterine fibroid embolization is not generally recommended for women who want to get pregnant, and a hysterectomy clearly rules out pregnancy.

MYOMECTOMY HISTORY

Myomectomy is the oldest known surgical treatment of fibroids and has been performed since the late 1800s. Its principal advantage is that it doesn't remove the uterus; its principal disadvantage is that fibroids may recur. A myomectomy may require a higher degree of surgical skill to perform than a hysterectomy, and some doctors do not recommend them or do not perform them, preferring the hysterectomy, which guarantees that fibroids are gone forever. Sadly, if your doctor does not know how to perform a myomectomy, he or she will probably not recommend that you have one, preferring to steer you toward something he or she can do.

We believed for years that when a woman was past her childbearing years, hysterectomy was the correct procedure for treating fibroids. We followed the prevailing medical logic that putting a woman through a surgery that doesn't cure her problem isn't worthwhile if she doesn't want any more children. "Why keep your uterus?" we would say, since its only known function in the body is incubating children. Over time it became clear to us that for many women, the uterus has value beyond its primary function. Many women we saw passionately voiced a desire to "die with all the organs they were born with," an idea we did not encounter in medical school. Because of this, we became more open to other surgical possibilities beyond the hysterectomy, even for women who do not "need" their uterus in the traditional medical sense of wanting to get pregnant.

We now fully appreciate something that may seem obvious: Only the woman herself, acting with the expert advice of her doctor, can decide what is right for her. For some women, hysterectomy with its guaranteed result will be the right choice. For others, keeping the body "whole" will be more important than facing the uncertain possibility of recurrence.

FIBROID RECURRENCE

Many women come to us with the impression that if they have a myomectomy their recurrence risk is close to 100 percent. A very careful analysis published in the journal *Human Reproduction Update* estimated the actual risk of recurrence. The authors calculated the chance that fibroids would come back using a statistical technique called life table analysis. This excellent paper provides the best look so far at how women have fared after myomectomy.

Overall, the authors found that the recurrence rate within five years after myomectomy varied from about 5 percent to just over 10 percent. This rate is based on the number of women who either needed surgery or had significant problems that were felt to be related to fibroids and had an ultrasound confirming that fibroids had recurred. Some studies that report a very high rate of recurrence include women who have had only ultrasound evidence of fibroids. Identifying fibroids on ultrasound doesn't mean much, as long as you feel fine; if you have no symptoms, then seeing fibroids on ultrasound should not affect your life.

On average, five to seven years go by after myomectomy before fibroids recur. The number of women who actually go on to have hysterectomy varies in different studies between 4 and 17 percent. Nowhere close to 100 percent, is it? Of course, the number of hysterectomies done will vary depending on how the women's gynecologists felt about performing second myomectomies. It certainly is possible to do second and even third myomectomies, but women who no longer want to have children will often be counseled to have a hysterectomy instead, since the scarring from previous surgery can make each subsequent myomectomy more difficult to perform.

Fibroid Recurrence

Studies of recurrence contribute to this confusion by the way the results are reported. The simplest studies merely report how many women out of a large group who had myomectomy ended up having more surgery after a certain number of years. The problem with this technique is that it ignores women who the authors knew nothing about by the end of the study. That is to say, if one hundred women started out with myomectomy and twenty were known to have recurrence and nothing is known about the other eighty, it might appear that the recurrence rate is twenty out of twenty.

In scientific literature, this problem is known as *ascertainment bias*. Ascertainment bias means that a condition can only be found in patients that you can see. The patients you can't see might be completely cured, and therefore not returning, or they could have gotten so much worse that they went somewhere else for care. The bottom line is that studies of this type are of little help in learning how likely you are to have a recurrence of fibroids after a myomectomy. (See also in chapter 4 the section "Infertility.")

Several factors will raise or lower the risk of recurrence after myomectomy, and you should consider these before deciding whether myomectomy, UFE, or hysterectomy is right for you. If you want to get pregnant, myomectomy is generally the best approach, and there is little point in worrying about the risk of recurrence or any other issue related to myomectomy. If you want a myomectomy to preserve your uterus but not because you want more children, then it's worth considering your chance of actually being able to avoid a hysterectomy in the long run.

Most studies have shown that younger women have a higher risk of recurrence after myomectomy. Women who have clinically significant fibroids at a younger age are more prone to rapid growth of fibroids than other women. Removing fibroids at myomectomy really only removes visible fibroids and there are undoubtedly many smaller, possibly even microscopic, fibroids left behind. As a result there is an increased risk of recurrence among younger women since they have undoubtedly more microscopic fibroids to begin with.

Women with multiple fibroids also have a higher risk of recurrence. Again, this might be because these women have many more microscopic fibroids, which can't be removed by surgery, and also because these same women might be prone to more rapid growth of fibroids.

As we touched on earlier, the use of GnRH agonists before myomectomy might increase the risk of recurrence since this treatment shrinks fibroids, and if fibroids shrink to a less than visible size, your surgeon won't be able to see them to remove them. Because GnRH agonists exert only a temporary effect, once the drug is withdrawn, those temporarily invisible fibroids may become visible once again.

It's too simple to say that this means that GnRH agonists

shouldn't be used before myomectomy. Other competing factors must be weighed as well. If using the drug will increase the likelihood of being able to make a low transverse incision instead of an up-and-down cut from belly button to pubic bone, or make laparoscopic surgery possible, or allow you to have a myomectomy without needing a blood transfusion, then using GnRH agonists might be worth the trade-off of a small increase in recurrence risk.

One key factor that affects fibroid recurrence is the method of surgery. Laparoscopic myomectomy seems to have a higher recurrence risk, with one study of 114 women published in 1998 showing that 51 percent had recurrent fibroids after five years.

Drug Treatment Prior to Fibroid Surgery

There are advantages and disadvantages to using GnRH agonists to shrink fibroids prior to surgery. The advantages of using these drugs include the following:

- Lessen anemia and bleeding and may reduce chance of transfusion
- May facilitate preferred forms of surgery, such as laparoscopic myoma resection
- May allow for a vaginal rather than abdominal hysterectomy in "borderline" cases
- May allow for a smaller "bikini" incision rather than a vertical incision
- May decrease blood loss during surgery
- May be necessary to "prepare" endometrium before hysteroscopy

Disadvantages:

- Surgeon may miss smaller fibroids
- May have unpleasant side effects
- End results are not necessarily better than surgery without drugs
- These drugs are expensive and not always covered by insurance

---

Perhaps even more important than how often fibroids recur after myomectomy is how well myomectomy works in the first place. Both the scientific literature and countless patients who have had the operation support our belief that myomectomy effectively relieves the symptoms of fibroids. Most studies have shown that over 90 percent of women have a resolution of their bleeding problems after myomectomy. Women who have pain as their primary symptom have a slightly lower chance of success, probably because one cannot be completely sure before surgery that fibroids are the cause of the pain. Pelvic pain can result from many different causes, and if fibroids are removed but other problems are not treated, the pain may not go away.

Women with so-called bulk symptoms—symptoms that are related to the pressure of a large uterus on the bladder, rectum, or other organs—are a group that has not been well studied as far as relief of symptoms after surgery. It makes sense, however, that if you make the uterus smaller by removing fibroids, these symptoms will go away. Similarly, there are very few studies of women whose primary complaint is urinary incontinence or other bladder problems and who are treated with myomectomy. We have clinically seen these women improve substantially, particularly if they had bladder testing before surgery that showed the fibroids to be the likely cause.

One major reason women have myomectomies is to preserve their ability to get pregnant. In fact, myomectomy has been used for many years as a treatment for infertility. Many different studies of fertility and pregnancy after myomectomy show that pregnancy occurs in about half of women who have myomectomy with the hope of restoring fertility. Unfortunately, this somewhat overstates the chance of a good outcome because many women will miscarry early in pregnancy. Most studies (and most surgeons) would prefer to report just the pregnancy rate since this makes the outcomes seem better. In reality, the pregnancy rate after myomectomy is probably about 50 percent lower than what is usually reported, meaning that about one in four women who have a myomectomy in order to get pregnant will be able to deliver a live infant. A 25 percent chance of getting pregnant should still be considered a good outcome since none of these women could get pregnant before they had surgery.

Women, particularly those over forty who do not want children, often hear, "You will be going through menopause in a few years, why not just have a hysterectomy?" But this is exactly the wrong attitude. It is precisely a woman like this, a forty-five-year-old not interested in having children, who has the greatest range of options. She can choose embolization or myomectomy, safe in the knowledge that, if fibroids don't recur by the time she hits menopause, she is "in the clear." Or she can choose hysterectomy and not have to worry about recurrence at all, but the choice is hers.

SURGICAL TECHNIQUE

Myomectomy is usually performed through a cut in the abdomen. The surgery takes from one to three hours, depending on the number and size of fibroids and their location and the type of surgery performed. Recovery usually involves a two- to three-day hospital stay, although with laparoscopic or hysteroscopic myomectomy, women can go home the same day they have surgery.

Abdominal Myomectomy

Abdominal myomectomy is usually the best type of myomectomy for women who want to have children because this method allows the uterus to be put back together in as close to a natural way as possible. In other types of myomectomy, such as laparoscopic myomectomy, the uterus cannot be sewn back together the same way. There have been reports of uterine rupture during pregnancy after laparoscopic myomectomy, and this is most likely a result of the inability to adequately repair the uterus. In an abdominal myomectomy, several layers of sutures are placed in the muscle of the uterus to secure it. In laparoscopic myomectomy, because the suturing is done using a long, narrow instrument, it is not as easy to repair the uterus in the same way.

Abdominal myomectomy involves a series of steps beginning with a cut in the abdominal wall. This cut is usually made at the bikini line and can be anywhere from three to six inches in length. After cutting through the skin, the surgeon moves through the various layers of tissue until reaching a strong fibrous layer of tissue called the fascia. This tissue is cut, usually in an incision that goes from side to side, paralleling the skin incision. After dividing the fascia, the surgeon will find the space between the sides of the abdominal muscles and enter the abdominal cavity. The surgeon will usually then feel around the abdomen and pelvis, making sure that there are no abnormalities other than the fibroids. If possible, the uterus is then gently elevated outside of the incision so it is almost lying on the abdomen. Surprisingly enough, the uterus is mobile enough in most cases that it can be lifted up and out of the pelvis in this way.

Once the uterus is easily accessible and it is clear that there are no other problems besides fibroids that need to be dealt with, the myomectomy begins. The basic principle of myomectomy is to make as few incisions on the uterus as possible while removing as many of the fibroids as possible. Sometimes there are only one or two fibroids and applying both of these principles is easy. Other times, there are literally dozens of small fibroids, and the surgeon has to make a decision about how many to remove while trying to minimize the number of incisions on the uterus. For women who are having myomectomy in order to be able to get pregnant, or who want to preserve the ability to get pregnant, one additional goal is to place the incisions on the uterus on the front or top rather than the back of the uterus. In the normal pelvis, the open ends of the fallopian tubes and the ovaries lie right behind the uterus. This is in contrast to many people's view of the ovaries as being somehow off to the sides. This image comes from photographs or drawings showing the uterus with the tubes and ovaries laid out next to the uterus. In the body, the fallopian tubes and ovaries, being mobile, tend to drop down into the space behind the uterus. When cuts are made on the back part of the uterus to remove fibroids, scarring from these cuts is more likely to block off the tubes, thereby making pregnancy more difficult. Sometimes incisions in this location are unavoidable, but it's not the preferred location.

When performing myomectomies to preserve fertility, surgeons will also try to avoid making cuts through the entire wall of the uterus into the cavity. This kind of "through and through" cut is thought to weaken the wall of the uterus more than an incision that only goes partway through the uterine muscle. Usually, a woman who has had a "through and through" cut is told that she will need to deliver by cesarean rather than normal labor. If the uterus has been weakened by this type of cut, the gynecologist worries that during labor the incision line could rip, causing the uterus to rupture.

After all the fibroids are removed and the uterus is sewn back together, it is replaced back through the incision. The surgeon carefully inspects the uterus to make sure there is no bleeding, and then closes the abdominal incision. Closing the abdomen usually involves sewing at least two layers of tissue. First, the fascial layer is sewn using a strong suture that will maintain its strength for at least a month. After this, the skin layer is closed using either a small suture that absorbs quickly or stainless steel staples.

After surgery, people sometimes wonder why it feels as though there is a hard lump or line running above where they can see the cut in their belly. This is because the fascial incision is not directly under the skin incision. Effectively, there are two different incisions, and you might feel one through the skin and be able to see the other on top of the skin.

Up to 15 percent of women need a blood transfusion during or immediately after surgery, as myomectomy can be a bloody process. As a precaution, some women donate a pint or two of their own blood in case a transfusion is necessary.

Some surgeons use drugs or special techniques during surgery to limit the loss of blood. The first technique is to use a chemical called vasopressin (Pitressin) to constrict the uterine blood vessels. Injected directly into the uterus right over the place where the surgeon is going to cut, vasopressin constricts the small blood vessels in the uterus, thereby reducing bleeding. The drug wears off after about twenty to thirty minutes. Some doctors worry about using this drug during surgery because they are afraid it will hide bleeding that will start up again once they've closed the abdomen. Studies have not supported this fear, however, and have shown that vasopressin reduces blood loss during myomectomy.

The second technique to reduce bleeding is to place a tourniquet, or very tight band, around the base of the uterus. This squeezes the uterine arteries during the operation, preventing blood from flowing to the uterus. Once the tourniquet is removed at the end of surgery, blood flow returns to normal. A final technique is to place temporary clamps, called vascular clamps, on the ovarian arteries, which supply blood to the ovaries and the uterus. Because the uterus is so richly supplied with blood, even putting clamps on the ovarian arteries and a tourniquet around the base of the uterus does not completely cut off the blood supply to the uterus. So even using all of these techniques does not entirely eliminate bleeding, but it does drastically reduce it.

Sometimes a surgeon planning a myomectomy will end up doing a hysterectomy because of excessive bleeding. Talk with the surgeon about this possibility before you make a decision about treatment. Some gynecologists make this intraoperative change of plans frequently, and some hardly ever do so. Given the availability of the techniques just described, we believe that less than 1 percent of myomectomies will need to convert to hysterectomies because of bleeding.

Complications other than bleeding include inadvertent damage to organs or parts of the body that lie close to the uterus, such as the bladder, intestines, ovaries, or ureters. These complications are very rare, happening in perhaps two or three out of a thousand surgeries.

Some complications don't occur until after surgery, including infection in the incision, pneumonia, or bladder infections. Most of these infections will occur while the woman is still in the hospital or shortly after discharge, and in most cases they are easily treated with antibiotics. Removing the bladder catheter within twenty-four hours of surgery reduces the risk of urinary tract infection. Shortly after surgery, women are often instructed to turn, cough, and breathe deeply while in bed. This clears the lungs and can help prevent pneumonia. Some doctors give antibiotics before surgery in order to reduce the risk of infection in the skin. This has never been shown to reduce infection in myomectomy, and since there are rare complications from giving antibiotics, we do not generally do this.

The most common long-term complication of myomectomy is the occurrence of internal scars, called adhesions. These scars can form between the uterus and the ovaries, fallopian tubes, intestines, or the inside of the pelvis. This is a fairly common occurrence after myomectomy and may be seen in up to 80 percent of women who have myomectomies, but probably fewer than one in ten of these women have problems related to these adhesions. In most cases, the adhesions sit quietly and are only noticed if surgery is performed again. In some cases, particularly if the adhesions that form are very thick and strong, they can cause pelvic pain. Also, if these adhesions form against the fallopian tubes, this can result in infertility.

Because of these potential complications, some surgeons use various techniques to reduce the risk of adhesion formation. The first technique is to carefully close the surface of the uterus after the fibroid has been removed, making sure that all bleeding on the surface of the uterus has been controlled. Sutures are chosen that will not cause too much inflammation, and they are placed in a particular way to reduce the risk of inflammation and possibly the risk of adhesion formation. Some surgeons use commercially available products to create a barrier over the uterus. These products are like sheets of paper that are laid across the uterus just before the abdomen is closed.

They dissolve slowly, but while they remain, they prevent scars from forming on the uterus. These barriers (Interceed is one of the most common) have been shown to reduce the risk of adhesions to about 30 percent. They are very expensive, however, so they are not always used unless fertility is a concern.

Energy Sources in Surgery

As you may remember from a high school physics class, energy means the ability to do work. When performing myomectomy, work must be done to remove the myomas, and the energy to do this work can come in many different forms. The simplest form is *physical energy* which of course is the surgeon's hand holding a scalpel and the scalpel cutting through the myoma tissue.

Although we don't commonly use it in gynecology, one could also use *chemical* energy to do work. Pouring some substance on a myoma that would cause it to burn up would be an example of chemical energy.

Electrical energy is commonly used in the operating room. A small device that looks almost like a pencil with a metal tip is a standard part of every operating room setup. This device, sometimes referred to by its trade name, Bovie, is used to both cut and stop bleeding in surgery. An electrical charge is delivered through the metal tip and, depending on the characteristics of the electricity, tissue that the tip of the instrument touches will either be cut, as with a knife, or coagulated, meaning that blood vessels within it will be "cooked" and stop bleeding.

Ultrasound energy is also used in the operating room, although less commonly than physical or electrical energy. To use ultrasound, a device similar to the Bovie but with a vibrating tip is placed near the tissue to be cut. The vibrations of the tip create sound waves that actually burn or cook the tissue the way electrical energy does.

Finally, there is the form of energy that is most exciting to the public imagination: laser. Laser is simply the use of coordinated light energy to perform the same tasks as any other energy source. Laser, which stands for *light amplification by the simulated emission of radiation*, was invented in 1957. Many of the common images of laser date from this time. We often picture laser as some type of a "space ray" or "death ray" that can deliver unlimited amounts of energy over great distances through a small beam of light. The truth of using laser in surgery is quite different from this. It works very much the same way as other energy sources.

The body's tissue responds to laser in a way that is essentially indistinguishable from its response to any other energy source. In some circumstances, laser is an ideal way to deliver energy to tissues. For example, when a Pap smear and biopsy show cervical abnormalities that might lead to cervical cancer, laser can be used to burn away part of the surface of the cervix. Similarly, laser can be perfect for burning away warts. What makes it ideal in these circumstances is that by adjusting the wavelength and strength of the laser, care can be taken to remove only the abnormalities and not the tissue underlying it, which sometimes lies only a few millimeters away. The disadvantages of laser are that it is expensive and generally slower than electrical or physical energy in making large incisions. During surgery for myomas, the laser might be used to cut the uterus that overlies the myoma, to stop bleeding, or to burn holes in the myoma with the hope of killing it.

While these applications of laser in gynecology are not unreasonable, there are no important advantages to using it over other sources of energy. Laser is too often used as a gimmick to draw women in to surgery. Because of the popular perception of laser as being some type of magical beam, women will often assume that surgery is the most high tech, least invasive, and best procedure possible. That's just not true. Saying that laser is going to be used in surgery should mean no more to you than being told that a knife is going to be used.

Choosing your doctor and choosing the surgery that you need is a process that requires consideration, thoughtfulness, and time. Focusing on catchwords will divert you from more important issues in making this crucial decision.

Laparoscopy

A laparoscope is a long, thin telescope that allows doctors to see inside your abdomen. Laparoscopic myomectomy can usually be done without requiring an overnight hospital stay, although it does require general anesthesia. The laparoscope is inserted through an incision near the naval. Two or three additional small incisions are made below the pubic hairline, and similarly thin instruments are inserted through these incisions to perform the surgery. The surgeon operates the small instruments with the aid of a video monitor. The fibroids are cut into small pieces, a process called *morcellation,* and the pieces are removed through tubes. Small scissors, lasers, radio waves, or ultrasound energy is used to open the uterus.

Laparoscopy is ideal for women with fibroids no larger than a few inches across that are located near the outside of the uterine wall. Compared to an abdominal myomectomy, laparoscopic surgery has several advantages including smaller incisions and smaller scars. The risk of infection is lower, and there is less pain after surgery. Women recover from laparoscopic myomectomy more rapidly than they do from open surgery, and most women can leave the hospital the same day they have surgery and return to work in a week or two.

Complications of laparoscopy are similar to those seen with open surgery, although the infection rate is lower. When the first instrument is put through the belly button incision, there is also a risk of poking it straight through the intestine. This uncommon complication can usually be dealt with quickly as long as it is noticed when it happens. The risk of this kind of accident is higher if the woman has had prior myomectomies or endometriosis, or has a history of pelvic infections.

Laparoscopic surgery is *not* recommended for women who want to get pregnant because there have been a few reports of women whose uterus eventually tears open during pregnancy after laparoscopic myomectomy. This may result because the uterus cannot be sutured or securely closed as well with miniature instruments operated from a distant location as it can be with stitches placed directly by hand. Another disadvantage when compared to open surgery is that the surgeon can't actually feel the fibroids with his or her fingers and might miss a small fibroid or two, making the recurrence rate higher. A third disadvantage to laparoscopic surgery is that it generally takes longer than open myomectomy, with some surgeries lasting as long as four or five hours.

Since laparoscopic myomectomy is relatively new and more technically demanding than abdominal myomectomy, it goes without saying that it should be done by a person certified and well trained in the use of the equipment. Large or numerous fibroids are more difficult to remove. Closing back the wall of the uterus from which fibroids have been removed is difficult to do well, and this is crucial if fertility is to be preserved. If you find a doctor who suggests this surgery, you should ask how many he or she has done successfully. While there is no magic number that makes someone capable, Dr. William Parker, author of *A Gynecologist's Second Opinion* and past president of the American Association of Gynecologic Laparoscopists, suggests that the procedure becomes much easier once the doctor has done at least twenty of them.

Hysteroscopy

If your fibroids are entirely submucosal and located entirely within the uterine cavity, a myomectomy may be performed by *hysteroscopic resection*. *Hysteroscopy* is useful particularly if these fibroids are causing abnormal bleeding or interfering with pregnancy.

The *hysteroscope* or *resectoscope* is a small telescope and video camera inserted into the uterus through the cervix that allows the doctor to view the inner surface of the uterus on a video monitor while performing surgery. No cutting is required in inserting these instruments because the cervix easily opens wide enough to allow the hysteroscope to pass through. Using a hysteroscope, it is a very easy procedure to remove fibroids attached to the inner lining of the uterus. To do so, a small amount of fluid is flushed through the uterus to expand it and allow the doctor to see the entire lining of the uterus. With the fluid swelling the uterus, a wire loop with electricity running through it is used to cut off the fibroid, either all at once or in sections if it is large. Depending on the skill of the surgeon, fibroids up to three centimeters in diameter may be removed in this way. The electricity in the wire loop stops any bleeding as it cuts, so the blood loss with hysteroscopy usually amounts to less than a few tablespoons.

Hysteroscopic resection can improve abnormal bleeding and remove fibroids that may be preventing pregnancy. An estimated 10 to 20 percent of women with fibroids who are bleeding are candidates for this procedure, and almost 90 percent of them will have normal periods after it's over. When fibroids are the cause of infertility, pregnancy rates in young, healthy women with no additional fertility problems are about 50 percent after this procedure, but much lower in older women.

Hysteroscopy is easier on the body than abdominal surgery since no incisions or cuts are made. Hysteroscopy causes very few serious complications, but fluid management can be tricky since too much fluid solution absorbed into the uterus can result in body chemistry problems. Doctors manage this by watching carefully how much fluid is used. Bleeding, infection, and injury to the uterus or other organs occur in fewer than two or three of every thousand cases. Not all physicians are trained to do it, so be sure your doctor has experience.

Before hysteroscopic surgery, your doctor might want to give you a treatment with Lupron or another GnRH agonist. The goal of this treatment is not really to shrink the fibroids but rather to thin the endometrial lining. This thinning reduces the amount of bleeding during the procedure and improves the surgeon's ability to remove fibroids or the endometrium successfully. Lupron has the effect of stopping the body's normal hormones so you might have symptoms of menopause. Usually, since only one month of Lupron is required before hysteroscopy, the symptoms are tolerable. If they're not, tell your doctor because medications are available to treat the symptoms. If you've had a bad reaction to Lupron in the past, or just don't want to use it, there are other ways to prepare the uterus for this surgery. Other GnRH agonists, or even birth control pills, can be used, although they are somewhat less effective. Discuss your options with your doctor before you plan any surgery of this type.

HOW TO PREPARE FOR SURGERY

Preparation for surgery may be very different depending on the type of procedure, whether the procedure will require you to stay in the hospital for several nights, or whether you'll be going home the day of the procedure. Your preparation might also vary depending on whether you'll be under general anesthesia or some type of regional anesthetic such as an epidural. For major abdominal surgery such as a myomectomy or hysterectomy, there are things that your doctor will do, things your anesthesiologist will do, and things you should do to prepare.

The anesthesiologist, the doctor who directs your anesthetic during surgery, will at a minimum have reviewed your record, know what type of procedure you're going to have, and have an idea of how long that procedure will take. He or she will also know about certain risk factors you may have. In particular, the anesthesiologist will focus on what other surgeries you may have had in the past and what type of anesthetic you had for those surgeries. The anesthesiologist is looking for possible bad reactions to anesthetic medications so he or she can avoid them. The anesthesiologist will also be very interested in any medications you are taking, including prescription, nonprescription, and herbs or supplements. Any of these types of medications may affect, for example, the way your blood clots or the way your body interacts with other drugs.

Preparing for Surgery

Things to do before you schedule surgery:

- Make sure you have all your questions answered about what exactly the surgery should accomplish.
- Ask how long you'll be in the hospital.
- Make sure you're comfortable with the doctor you've selected and the hospital in which you'll be having your procedure.
- Make sure you're honest with your anesthesiologist and tell him or her about every medication you are taking even if you don't take it on a daily basis.

For some types of gynecologic surgery, and depending on your general overall health, the anesthesiologist may get all the information he or she needs from reviewing your records, examining lab reports, and possibly talking to you briefly over the telephone. In any case, you will be required to come to an office for a "preop visit." At this visit you may have blood taken, have a physical exam, or undergo other tests or procedures. The most common preoperative tests besides blood tests include EKG to examine your heart and look for evidence of previous heart attacks, and chest X rays to examine your lungs. Whether you will need any of these procedures will depend on the surgery that is planned, your age and anesthetic risk factors, and sometimes the protocol or rules of the hospital.

Preparation for outpatient surgery usually requires far less involvement by the anesthesiologist. Outpatient procedures generally have lower risk and therefore do not require the same intensive level of scrutiny. For these procedures, your contact with the anesthesiologist may be limited to several minutes before the procedure begins. Regardless of the manner in which this interaction occurs, it is crucial that you be entirely open and honest with the anesthesiologist before surgery. For example, if you are instructed not to take Motrin or aspirin before surgery and you inadvertently do so, you must tell the doctor about this. It will do you no good, and may do you a world of harm, if, in your embarrassment, you are not completely truthful. Be frank and honest with your doctors so they can make the best decisions about whether to proceed with your surgery.

Your preparation for surgery will have a number of components. First, you need to prepare psychologically. Depending on the type of procedure, this may involve nothing more than taking off work for a day or so and making sure you have somebody to drive you home. For major abdominal surgery such as myomectomy or hysterectomy, you need to consider what it will mean not to be able to engage in most of your usual activities for a month or more. Consider very carefully how it will affect your life not to be able to climb stairs, drive a car, or perhaps even prepare your own meals temporarily. It's not necessary to be scared by these preparations, but you should think about them when planning your surgery. People with seasonal employment, for example, may want to plan their surgery for a time when work is less hectic. When symptoms are very severe, however, this type of planning may not be possible.

You must also prepare physically for your surgery. Again, depending on how much time you have to make the decision and to plan your surgery, and the nature of the procedure, this physical preparation can take different forms. Even for relatively minor outpatient procedures, you should be sure to get adequate rest in the weeks leading up to the procedure. Surgery is a stressful experience, one that your body can handle better if well rested. If you are particularly anxious and are afraid you won't be able to sleep in the nights before your procedure, ask your doctor for a prescription sleeping medication to use in the short term before surgery. You won't get addicted, and it may help you go into your operation better prepared. In the short run, there is little a change in diet can do to prepare you for surgery with the exception of combating anemia. If you are anemic and have been instructed by your doctor to take iron or eat iron-rich foods, you should do so exactly as instructed. While the risks of blood transfusion have been dramatically lowered by advanced testing of blood products, it is certainly better to avoid transfusion when possible, and having a higher blood count can help you do this. We discussed iron supplements and iron-containing foods in chapter 6.

Personal Preparation

- Get plenty of sleep in the weeks leading up to surgery.
- Make sure you follow your doctor's advice about diet or medications to take before surgery.
- Don't bring valuables to the hospital.
- Wear glasses, not contact lenses.
- Wear loose-fitting clothing.
- For outpatient surgery, arrange a ride.
- For longer stays, arrange for someone to check your mail and stop newspaper delivery.
- Bring a portable music player with headphones.

If you have a long period of time to prepare for surgery and are feeling well, then increasing your level of physical fitness can make your recovery dramatically easier. Women who are physically fit tolerate surgery more easily and recover more quickly than more sedentary women. Even though during surgery you are paralyzed and asleep, surgery is like an intense bout of exercise, like a marathon. It is a strain on your body, and if your body has over time developed a tolerance to such strains by regular exercise, surgery will be easier to withstand.

Finally, there are the mechanical preparations for surgery. Again, how much preparation you will need depends on what type of procedure you're having and how long you may be spending in the hospital. If you're having an outpatient procedure, you may just need to prepare to have someone to drive you home and remember to wear loose-fitting clothing to the hospital. (This is a good idea so that tight or binding clothes don't press on sensitive incision sites.) You should definitely not bring any jewelry to the hospital. If you do, the hospital staff will do their best to secure your belongings, but they are certainly safer at home. If you wear contact lenses, you should generally leave them out and wear your glasses instead, unless instructed otherwise by your anesthesiologist. Most anesthesiologists prefer that you not wear nail polish when you're having surgery. The beds of the nails can indicate how well the small blood vessels in your body are filled with blood. Also oxygen monitors that fit over your fingertip can be fooled by opaque nail polish.

If you wear dentures, you will generally be asked to remove them for surgery. If you're self-conscious about not having your dentures, you can certainly wear them to the hospital, but be sure to remove them and give them to the hospital staff before you're taken to the operating room. Loose-fitting denture can make it extremely difficult to place a breathing tube which may be crucial to your receiving adequate oxygen during the surgery.

If your surgery will require you to spend more than a few hours in the hospital, you may want to bring a portable CD or tape player. Some studies have shown that people listening to the music of their choice after surgery have less severe pain than those who cannot listen to music. As a side benefit, a portable music player may allow you to tune out a noisy roommate or bothersome hospital noise.

POSTOPERATIVE CARE

If you have had abdominal surgery, your doctor will usually want to see you back in the office two to six weeks after the surgery. In the time after you're released from the hospital and before you see the doctor, you might notice some gradual changes in your body. First, your need for pain medication will probably decrease gradually, and your activity level will gradually increase. But even though you're generally getting better, some things might seem not to be changing. For example, there is often quite a bit of swelling around an incision. This swelling can take months to disappear. Particularly in the area above and below a low transverse incision, this swelling can be quite noticeable and sometimes bothersome. The swelling usually doesn't represent a problem.

Under some circumstances you should call your doctor to confirm that things are going okay. First, if the swelling around the incision seems to be getting worse and not better, this may be a sign of an infection, and you should probably call your doctor. If the area around the incision is turning red or pink or becomes increasingly sensitive to touch, this also might be an early warning sign of infection. Finally, if a thick yellow or foul-smelling fluid is escaping from the incision, you should definitely call your doctor. Sometimes a clear or yellow-colored fluid will ooze out of an incision; while this is usually not a sign of infection, you should still communicate it to your doctor. Infections of an incision happen most commonly in the first week or two after surgery, but if these warning signs happen even after the first two weeks, you should still bring them to your doctor's attention.

Even if everything goes well and you have no infection, you still may have some unusual sensations as you heal. One of the most common postoperative complaints after a low transverse incision is the sensation of numbness, tingling, or even burning in the area above and below the incision. During surgery, the small nerves in the skin are cut. These nerves do regrow, but they do so very slowly, sometimes requiring as much as six months to a year before they are fully healed. During this time, you may feel a tingling or numbness extending upward from the incision. This area may reach as high as your belly button. Rest assured that these sensations will resolve slowly.

In very unusual cases, a nerve in the skin can be injured during surgery and not heal normally. In this case, pain or abnormal feelings may persist long after surgery. These cases are unusual and may often be treated with several injections of local anesthetic into the bothersome areas. These injections serve to quiet the nerves while normal function is restored.

Another common question in the postoperative period involves the way the incision itself feels as it heals. Within a week or two after surgery, the scar itself might begin to feel thick and firm. This is a normal part of the healing process. Over time this scar will become softer, but it can take up to a year before the scar reaches the stage at which it will remain for the rest of your life. This thickening of the scar represents new tissue that is being formed and is your body's way of protecting the injured area. As the scar thickens and heals, it might retract or pull downward. This can be felt by running your hand along the scar. You might feel a slight ditch in your abdomen. Again, this is a normal occurrence and will resolve gradually as the scar softens.

Women also sometimes notice another ridge of thick tissue slightly above the scar and under the skin. They may also notice firm knots at either end of the incision. To understand these things, you have to understand a little bit about the anatomy of the abdominal wall and the process of making a surgical incision.

The abdominal wall consists of several layers that are only loosely attached, like the way a bed might be covered by a bedspread, a blanket, and a sheet. If you were to try to cut through these layers down to the mattress, you could cut directly through all the layers in one fell swoop, or cut each one individually. During surgery, the surgeon is careful to cut each layer individually so that he or she can repair it carefully at the end of surgery.

In order to make the skin incision cosmetically appealing, the surgeon usually cuts the skin just below the top of the pubic hairline. This location isn't always the most convenient place to cut through the thick layer of tissue (the fascia) that helps to hold your abdominal contents in place. This incision on the fascia is often made as much as an inch above where the skin incision was placed. This fascial incision may also be larger than the skin incision.

Particularly in thin women, the fascial incision can be felt by placing your hand above the skin incision and gently pressing downward. This incision thickens in the same way that the skin incision does. As the thickening becomes more pronounced, it might become noticeable with gentle pressure on your belly. The lumps that can sometimes be felt on either end of the incision usually represent areas where the suture was tied when the incision on the fascia was closed. This incision will often in the same way that the skin incision does and will not be noticeable within three to six months after surgery.

Not much can be done about these postoperative changes in your body. They will resolve with time, and as long as they don't represent worrisome things such as infection, they generally don't need to be treated. In some cases, continuing to take an anti-inflammatory drug such as ibuprofen (Motrin) will reduce the swelling that you may notice around the incision. Some people believe that rubbing vitamin E or other creams into the incision will help the wound soften, but there is very little evidence to support this belief.

Some scars will form keloids, thick, overgrown scars that can form anywhere the skin is injured. While African American women are more prone to this type of scarring, it can happen to anyone. Cells in a keloid scar don't stop growing the way cells in a normal scar do, and as a result the scar becomes thick and can protrude above the surface of the skin.

Controlling keloid formation is a hotly debated topic in the medical literature, primarily because there is little good research to suggest any effective ways of stopping keloids from forming. Some practitioners try to inject steroids into the incision in the hope that this will reduce the inflammation and perhaps reduce keloiding. It is not clear that this method works very well, however, and steroids can have a downside, causing collapse of the tissue under the scar. This collapse can lead to a cosmetically unappealing scar that dips beneath the surface of the skin.

Keloids are more likely to form when there is poor healing. As a result, techniques that improve wound healing should probably be routinely employed. This includes careful, layer by layer closure of the incision, care taken that all surgical bleeding is stopped, and an attempt to reduce the amount of foreign material in the incision. The surgeon should use the least amount of suture and the smallest suture possible.

How do you know if you will get keloids? If you have never had surgery or significant injury, it may not be possible to know if you're at risk for keloid formation. On the other hand, some women develop such severe keloids and with such little provocation that even the act of piercing the ears can cause massive keloids to form. For women like this, keloiding can become a major problem and may even lead them to avoid surgery that they would otherwise undergo. If you are African American, or have had prior keloids develop, you should discuss the issue with your doctor before surgery. There is some evidence that sutures that go through the skin are more likely to produce keloids than those under the skin. Ask your doctor whether he or she plans to use a subcuticular closure, which doesn't involve sutures going through the skin. You may also want to avoid the use of surgical staples, which travel through the skin.

Once a keloid scar has formed, there may be little that can be done about it. Sometimes surgery is attempted to remove the keloid tissue. Of course, since any type of surgery can produce a keloid, surgical removal may just substitute a new scar for the old one.

CONTINUED PROBLEMS AFTER SURGERY

While the success rate for myomectomy in improving bleeding and pain from fibroids is very high, not everybody is cured by this operation. Sometimes in the first few months after surgery, your periods may continue to be very heavy and unpredictable. It may take as long as three months for this bleeding to stabilize. Just as there are scars on the outside of your abdomen where the incision was made, there are scars on your uterus as well. Some of these scars may continue to leak a small amount of blood into the uterine cavity, which can then be seen as vaginal bleeding. In addition, your body's precise hormonal balance can be thrown off by the stress of surgery, altering your normal menstrual cycle.

If after three months your bleeding has not normalized, you should see your doctor again. (Of course, this only applies if you've had a myomectomy; if you've had a hysterectomy, any bleeding other than a few small spots after surgery is abnormal.) If myomectomy doesn't cure bleeding, there are a variety of explanations. First, a small fibroid may have been missed during the surgery. To guard against this possibility or to establish whether this is the case, your doctor may want to obtain an ultrasound or MRI if your bleeding persists.

Persistent bleeding after myomectomy may also occur because the fibroids were never the problem to begin with. Sometimes a woman with a completely normal uterus will have abnormal, heavy, persistent bleeding unrelated to fibroids. Since fibroids are common, she may also have several fibroids. Her doctor may assume that the fibroids are responsible for the bleeding, but they may just be innocent bystanders. Removing the fibroids may not have any permanent effect on bleeding. Unfortunately, little can be done to predict this in advance, but using noninvasive treatments before turning to surgery will reduce this risk.

If the bleeding persists and a fibroid left behind is ruled out as a possibility, you must consider your options once again. Usually, at this point a renewed evaluation for other possible causes of bleeding will begin. Many of these evaluations should be done routinely before any surgery takes place, but it is certainly a good idea to repeat them if the myomectomy doesn't solve the problem. Specifically, your doctor may want to sample the endometrium again with an endometrial biopsy. He or she may also want to check for evidence of bleeding disorders or problems with blood clotting. You may also need to be evaluated for disturbances or abnormalities in the hormonal system, for example, hyper- or hypothyroidism.

Pain sometimes persists after surgery as well. In other cases, pain may resolve immediately after surgery only to recur several months later. Pain is a poorly understood phenomenon, and sometimes recurrent pain after surgery is never fully explainable. In other cases, once an explanation can be found, the appropriate treatment can be instituted, and the pain can be relieved. In a very small percentage of women who have abdominal surgery, pain develops at the site of the skin incision when a nerve becomes trapped by scar tissue. The brain interprets the signals sent by the trapped nerve as pain, although nothing "painful" is going on. To understand how this might happen, you need to understand something about how pain is perceived in the body.

Scientists sometimes say that all sensation takes place in the brain. Nerves send electrical impulses along their length to the brain. How the brain understands these impulses determines whether the stimulus is felt as pleasurable, painful, or somewhere between the two. Pain is usually thought to be a warning sign so that, for example, when you touch a hot surface, the pain tells your brain to tell your hand to move. In some cases, these signals can become confused, and the nerve may send a signal that is interpreted as pain but is just a normal, everyday touch. This "misinterpretation" can cause pain that doesn't respond to the usual treatments.

When nerve entrapment causes pain, injections of local anesthetic or sometimes just sterile water can relieve the pain. It is thought that these injections temporarily calm the signal from the nerve long enough for the brain to interpret the information properly. At other times, the solution is not so straightforward. It may be thought, for example, that pelvic pain results from uterine fibroids. If the fibroids are removed and the pain persists, consideration must be given to other possible causes of the pain. A thorough preoperative workup followed by an attempt to control pain nonsurgically can help ensure that the proposed procedure, whether it is myomectomy or hysterectomy, will relieve the pain.

A generalized feeling of fullness in the pelvis or pain when a hand is pressed onto the uterus through the abdominal wall can be fairly reliably explained as coming from uterine fibroids. Similarly, pain that occurs at the time of menses in the presence of fibroids inside the cavity of the uterus is another situation in which the pain and the fibroids are very likely to be linked. In other circumstances—for example, when sharp pelvic pain occurs sporadically but not in relation to the menstrual cycle—it is harder to be sure that fibroids are responsible. In a circumstance such as this, a diagnostic laparoscopy, in which a surgeon looks into the abdomen for any other possible causes of pain, is a reasonable option before proceeding to more invasive surgery. The goal of a thorough preoperative evaluation and treatment plan is to ensure that only people who are likely to benefit from surgery get it.

Of course, it is not possible to guarantee a result simply because none of these diagnostic tests are perfect. The best way to be sure that any treatment plan is a successful one is to follow a carefully thought out and individualized plan. Such a plan can only be established by the doctor and patient working together.

Questions to Ask Your Surgeon

- Are you board certified, with advanced training in the treatment you plan to employ, such as laser surgery, laparoscopy, or hysteroscopy?
- What is your philosophy regarding preserving the uterus?
- How many surgeries of this type have you performed?
- How many of your surgeries have resulted in complications?
- How many of your myomectomies have turned into hysterectomies?

CHOOSING A DOCTOR

Patients often wonder how they can be sure their doctor "knows what he's doing." The truth is, it is difficult to find any independent way to be assured of this. There are some things you can do, however. First, confirm that your doctor is board certified in obstetrics and gynecology. Board certification means that your doctor has finished medical school and a residency in obstetrics and gynecology and has been in practice for at least two years. The doctor then must undergo an in-person examination by a panel of examiners who ask questions about gynecology practice. Only after passing this exam can a doctor advertise him- or herself as being board certified. Don't assume that your doctor is board certified because he or she has been in practice for many years or has admitting privileges at a nearby hospital. In order to practice medicine in most states, a doctor must graduate from medical school and have a medical license, which can be obtained after one year of post–medical school training. Board certification in obstetrics and gynecology is not possible without at least four years of post–medical school training. Unfortunately, board certification doesn't guarantee high quality. Think of it simply as a minimum standard that should be met.

Doctors performing gynecologic surgery may obtain certification through other programs or societies. Those with additional training, specifically in dealing with cancers of the reproductive system, may become board certified in oncology. This generally means that they have had at least three more years of training in complicated gynecologic surgery and care of women with cancer. Another society that certifies gynecologists is the American Association of Gynecologic Laparoscopists (AAGL). Membership in this society requires that the doctor perform a certain number of laparoscopic procedures and meet educational requirements. Again, neither of these certifications indicates that the doctor is using good judgment or is a good surgeon.

What else can you do to make sure your doctor is qualified? First, talk to women this doctor has taken care of in the past. While you obviously can't talk to all of his or her patients, you should be able to at least get a sense of whether they were satisfied with the care they received. Second, each state has a way that you can check for actions by the state medical board against a particular physician. In many states this information is available over the Internet.

At some point you just have to trust your gut instinct when choosing a doctor. Do you feel comfortable with this doctor? Is he or she answering your questions to your satisfaction? Do you feel that he or she is paying attention to you as an individual?

The Quality of Surgical Care in the United States

Despite the fact that 41 million Americans each year have major surgery, remarkably little is known about the overall quality of the surgical care these people receive. We conducted a study in 2001 examining what patients could learn about the quality of the surgical care they were about to have. At least five organizations, including government-funded organizations, private for-profit organizations, and nonprofit organizations, publicly release information about the quality of surgical care in the United States.

These organizations currently release information in two general areas. First, they collect and release information on how many of certain types of procedures are performed in a given hospital. For example, you can learn how many coronary bypass surgeries are performed every year in almost any hospital in the United States. You can't learn how many hysterectomies, myomectomies, or other gynecologic surgeries are performed because no organizations publicly report this information.

For some procedures, such as back surgery or heart valve replacements, you can learn how often patients die in the hospital after surgery. Again, there are no such numbers released for gynecologic surgery. Lest you think that gynecology is being ignored on purpose, realize that only three hundred thousand of the 41 million operations done each year have any publicly available quality information related to them. That means that 87 percent of the people who have surgery each year in the United States will not be able to find any information on the quality of the care they are going to have.

The field of quality measurement in surgery is really in its infancy; ten years ago, most of the measures described in the previous paragraph had not even been considered. In the next ten years measures of other kinds of surgery may be publicly released. Political pressure from women's groups and the support of gynecologists will both be necessary before meaningful quality information on specific gynecologic surgeries becomes available.

In the meantime, how should you choose your doctor? First, choose a doctor that is board certified in obstetrics and gynecology. Second, find a doctor whose patients speak highly of him or her. Third, try to find a doctor at an academic medical center or, if there is not one nearby, at a center that trains residents in obstetrics and gynecology. These types of hospitals tend to be more involved in leading edge research, and doctors there may be more aware of newer techniques.

Finally, you should consider a doctor who practices on the faculty of an academic medical center or a hospital that trains residents in obstetrics and gynecology. Physicians at these centers tend to keep up with the latest advances. (Of course, doctors practicing side by side in the same medical center can have varying skills and opinions.) Also, having resident and medical students involved in your surgery may be advantageous. Although it might be bothersome to have medical students and residents asking you so many questions, some studies have shown the quality of care at teaching hospitals to be superior to that of other hospitals.

GOOD CHOICES

Myomectomy is an invasive surgical procedure that removes fibroids but doesn't remove the uterus. It has advantages and disadvantages for women with fibroids. The greatest risk is that fibroids can grow back, but this only happens in a minority of cases. Myomectomy is the best choice for women who need invasive treatment and want to still be able to get pregnant. While abdominal myomectomy is still the most frequently performed kind of myomectomy, new forms of surgery including laparoscopic surgery and hysteroscopy are suitable for women whose fibroids are in particular locations. Myolysis and endometrial ablation are other choices to treat fibroids (see chapter 14). The most common surgery performed for fibroids, the hysterectomy, is covered in the next chapter.

Chapter 13

Hysterectomy

The word *hysterectomy* strikes terror into the hearts of many women, but it is a relatively safe operation with a 150-year track record of relieving symptoms related to fibroids. Hysterectomy can be a reasonable option to consider if you need surgery for fibroids. The key thing to remember is that it is an option—there are other choices. Hysterectomy is a life-saving procedure for some women with fibroids, and a good choice for many women seeking guaranteed, permanent relief from fibroid symptoms. Hysterectomies are performed through incisions in the abdomen or in the vagina. Although complications can occur, the great majority of women who have had hysterectomies are satisfied with the results and are happy to have fibroids gone once and for all.

The American College of Obstetricians and Gynecologists recommends several options for the treatment of fibroids but states that hysterectomy remains the most common treatment because "it is the only treatment that provides a cure and eliminates the possibility of recurrence." Hysterectomy can be the best option for women with unbearable symptoms who want no more children and who don't want to take the chance that another surgery or invasive procedure for fibroids will be needed at a later time.

Hysterectomy rates are extremely high in the United States compared with many other developed countries, and we believe that is largely because gynecologists recommend hysterectomy as the only option without trying other things first. Hysterectomy does get rid of fibroids, but many women could get by with less radical procedures. The author of *Sex, Lies, and the Truth about Uterine Fibroids*, Carla Dionne, puts it very clearly: "Women are being presented with the idea of having a hysterectomy in ways that they believe they *have* to have it. Yet, the procedure is always documented as though the woman had made that choice. Remember that hysterectomy is *elective*. Elective means it's a choice between options."

Dionne advises women with fibroids to educate themselves as to what tests they need and what procedures are available, to get copies of their medical reports, and to make informed decisions regarding their own health care. "I am an advocate of educating yourself. No physician is ever going to live in your body," Dionne tells women. "You have the greatest vested interest in your survival and the quality of your life."

Currently, more than half a million American women every year have hysterectomies, most commonly to remove fibroids. About half of these surgeries are done on women under forty.

OVERUSE OF HYSTERECTOMY

Five decades of science have shown that too many hysterectomies are done with too little justification. In 1947 a study showed that many surgeons performing hysterectomies to treat uterine fibroids found no fibroids at the time of surgery. A study in 1956 also found that many hysterectomies could not be justified based on the findings at the time of surgery or notes written in the medical record. In the 1980s concern with high levels of hysterectomy led a group of doctors in Switzerland to begin a mass education campaign about reducing the rate of hysterectomy. They found that by educating doctors and patients about options, the hysterectomy rate could safely be reduced. A study in the United States in the early 1990s continued to show that as many as 15 percent of hysterectomies were done without adequate justification. This study, written by Dr. Steven Bernstein and published in the *Journal of the American Medical Association*, showed that many women had hysterectomies even when they had minimal symptoms.

In the late 1990s we performed a study subsequently published in the journal of *Obstetrics and Gynecology* in 2000. We studied close to five hundred women at nine separate medical groups in Southern California. Fifty years after the first published study showing that many hysterectomies were done with too little justification, we found that 14 percent of the women we studied should probably never have had a hysterectomy. Medical records stated that these women had had surgery for pelvic pain or prolapse of the uterus, but when we interviewed these women, they denied ever having these problems. Perhaps even more concerning, 70 percent of the women we studied had not had an adequate workup before surgery, or they were not treated with less invasive therapy before surgery. That is, seven out of ten women with abnormal bleeding had not had a simple test to rule out cancer before they were taken for surgery. Many of the women who had had hysterectomies for pelvic pain had not been treated with simple, low-risk medications such as ibuprofen or did not have the proper investigations into the cause of their pain (such as laparoscopy to make sure that conditions such as endometriosis weren't responsible).

The gynecologists in our study were not bad doctors and certainly did not want to hurt their patients, but they jumped to treat common gynecologic problems with overly invasive solutions. Study after study has shown that the vast majority of women who have hysterectomies are happy with the results, and the patients in our study were no different. But there are compelling reasons to believe that many of the women who are satisfied with hysterectomies would probably have been satisfied with less invasive surgery or perhaps with no surgery at all.

Gynecologists overuse hysterectomy because it is safe and it works. More than 90 percent of women with pelvic pain who have hysterectomy are cured, and women who have bleeding problems before surgery have no bleeding afterward. The serious complication rate from hysterectomy is very low. Doctors are treating women with a procedure that works; they have very little incentive to change their practices. Patient education and a more thorough discussion of all the options are probably the only ways that the hysterectomy rate in this country will drop. The education campaign carried out in Switzerland in the 1980s produced about a 25 percent drop in the rate of hysterectomy. If this were repeated in the United States, it might mean 150,000 fewer hysterectomies every year!

APPROACHES TO HYSTERECTOMY

There are several ways for your doctor to do a hysterectomy. The most common way, accounting for three-quarters of all hysterectomies in the United States, is the *total abdominal hysterectomy.* In this procedure, the entire uterus is removed through a cut in the abdomen. A *total vaginal hysterectomy* means removing the uterus through the vagina. Contrary to popular belief, "total hysterectomy" does not mean that the ovaries are removed, but simply that the entire uterus is taken out. This is in contrast to a "partial hysterectomy" (more correctly called a supracervical hysterectomy), in which the cervix, or opening to the uterus, is left in place. *Oophorectomy* means removal of the ovaries, while *salpingo-oophorectomy* means removing the ovaries and fallopian tubes.

Medical Acronyms

TAH	Total abdominal hysterectomy
VH	Vaginal hysterectomy
LH	Laparoscopic hysterectomy
LAVH	Laparoscopically assisted vaginal hysterectomy
LSO	Removal of left ovary and fallopian tube
RSO	Removal of right ovary and fallopian tube
BSO	Removal of both ovaries and fallopian tubes
TAH/BSO	Total abdominal hysterectomy with removal of both ovaries and fallopian tubes

About 25 percent of hysterectomies are performed through an incision in the vagina. Vaginal hysterectomies have fewer complications and a shorter recovery period, are less expensive, and result in shorter hospital stays—about a day less than abdominal hysterectomy on average, according to a study published in the *New England Journal of Medicine*. Why aren't they all done this way? Well, vaginal hysterectomy may be difficult if the uterus is very large (more than the size of a twelve-week pregnancy) or if you've never delivered a child vaginally (because the vagina is smaller). Experienced surgeons can often perform vaginal surgery even in these circumstances, however, so if you have decided on hysterectomy, it is worth trying to find a gynecologist with experience in these difficult cases who might be able to do a vaginal, rather than abdominal, hysterectomy.

Vaginal hysterectomies are sometimes performed with the aid of laparoscopy, using miniature instruments mounted on tubes. This technique may allow a vaginal hysterectomy even in the case of a large uterus. Practice makes perfect with this technique, so if your doctor recommends it, make sure he or she has done at least twenty.

Laparoscopic Hysterectomy

In a true laparoscopic hysterectomy, no incision is made in the vagina. Instead, only laparoscopic instruments are used; they are placed through three to four incisions in the abdomen, each less than an inch long. In this procedure the entire hysterectomy is performed through these laparoscopic instruments, and then, because the uterus is too large to be taken out through a one-inch incision, it is *morcellated*, or cut up in small pieces, and removed through the small incisions. Because this morcellation process is slow, the bigger the uterus is, the longer the procedure takes. Since a uterus filled with fibroids can take hours to cut into small pieces, this technique is not commonly used for women with fibroids. Laparoscopic hysterectomy accounts for less than one out of every hundred hysterectomies done in this country.

Removing Ovaries

It is a common misconception that ovaries and the cervix are *always* removed during a hysterectomy. The ovaries are removed in nearly three-fourths of all hysterectomies performed in the United States, but it is rarely necessary for women with fibroids to have this done. One medical term for removing ovaries is *castration*—a term we usually associate with removing testicles, but which really means removing sex glands, either testicles or ovaries. This term strikes fear in the hearts of men. Women should also take it very seriously. Removing your ovaries throws the body into instant menopause with all the attendant symptoms. Hysterectomy on its own does not cause immediate menopause, even though periods stop.

Hysterectomy and Menopause

For a woman with a uterus, menopause occurs when menstruation stops. This is because ovarian production of estrogen progressively declines and the endometrium thins. A thin endometrium cannot bleed enough to cause a period. If your uterus is removed, but your ovaries continue to produce estrogen and progesterone, you are not really in menopause despite the lack of periods. Many women in this situation can still "feel" themselves ovulate, and they do not get hot flashes or other menopausal symptoms.

Vicky, a fifty-six-year-old dental assistant, was advised by her gynecologist to have a hysterectomy about a year ago. Vicky had suffered heavy menstrual bleeding for years. The heavy bleeding became so severe that Vicky went through four super tampons at her high school reunion, and still leaked through to her shorts.

Vicky was not offered any alternatives to hysterectomy by her doctor. She did not know when her mother or grandmother entered menopause since they both had hysterectomies too.

"I can take your ovaries now, or I can see you back in ten years and take them out then," Vicky's gynecologist told her. Given this choice, Vicky elected to have her ovaries and uterus removed.

The hysterectomy went smoothly, and Vicky recovered quickly from the operation. One year later Vicky is on supplemental estrogen to alleviate severe hot flashes.

According to the U.S. Centers for Disease Control and Prevention, well over half of the women who have hysterectomies in the United States also have their ovaries removed. The older the woman is, the more likely the doctor is to recommend that she have her ovaries removed. Doctors sometimes argue that removing the ovaries can prevent ovarian cancer, but the risk of testicular cancer doesn't have men lining up to have their testicles removed.

In 1965 only 25 percent of women who had hysterectomies had their ovaries removed. By 1984 that figure had increased to 41 percent. By 1993, 52 percent of women having a hysterectomy had their ovaries removed, and the numbers continue to rise. Doctors' and patients' desire to prevent ovarian cancer is probably the driving force behind this trend, but the argument that "you might get cancer later so why not get rid of your ovaries now?" is just too simplistic.

When your ovaries are removed, you experience an instant, surgically created menopause. Symptoms of menopause such as hot flashes and vaginal dryness are usually then treated with estrogen and this may bring with it a new set of problems. The risk of heart attacks and osteoporosis increases *significantly* when the ovaries are removed; both of these diseases are much more common and kill many more women than ovarian cancer. Some studies have shown that a thirty-five-year-old woman who has her ovaries removed has a seven times greater chance of having a heart attack or heart problems than the average woman!

Women who have undergone surgical menopause lose bone twice as fast as women whose menopause is natural, and this bone loss is more severe in women whose ovaries have been removed before the age of thirty-five. You can lower your risk of osteoporosis with hormone replacement, but hormone pills are not the same as natural hormones. You will find very few men standing in line to have their testicles removed just because synthetic testosterone pills exist. Doctors don't recommend having your thyroid gland removed to prevent thyroid cancer, even though thyroid replacement hormone is cheap and easy to take.

In the general population, ovarian cancer occurs in about one in every seventy women. Some women are at much higher risk. If you have both a mother and a sister who had ovarian cancer, your chances of contracting ovarian cancer are almost fifty-fifty. (The risk of women with a certain genetic marker for cancer may be this high as well.) With two second-degree relatives, such as aunts or cousins, your chance of getting ovarian cancer is one in four—much higher than average and you may want to consider having your ovaries removed if your risk is this high.

Strangely enough, even removing your ovaries doesn't guarantee that ovarian cancer will not occur. Although it is rare, ovarian cancer has been diagnosed in women whose ovaries have been removed since it can spread microscopically to areas away from the ovaries before they are removed, and small amounts of ovarian-type tissue exist outside the ovaries.

Taking out normal ovaries during surgery for fibroids is generally a bad decision. Unless the surgeon notices a serious problem during the surgery, or you have a strong family history of ovarian cancer or a genetic marker for ovarian cancer, the risks of surgical castration probably outweigh the benefits. Each situation is unique, however, so discuss plans for removing your ovaries with your doctor before surgery. Don't accept the statement that "you're not using them anyway" as an explanation. Body parts are not disposable. Ovaries continue functioning and producing hormones well beyond menopause.

Removing the Cervix

Unless you have a history of cervical cancer or precancer, it is not necessary to remove the cervix when you are having a hysterectomy for fibroids. An important bundle of nerves called the *uterovaginal plexus* has branches in the cervix. These nerves may be important in sexual function, particularly in women who experience orgasm in the uterus (uterine orgasm). A research study from Finland gave some evidence that women experience more sexual pleasure if the cervix is not removed.

Surgically removing the cervix can also shorten the vagina, which can reduce sexual enjoyment Removing the cervix may place you at greater risk for stress incontinence, although again, this is not well studied. Within the abdomen, the cervix helps keep the floor of the pelvis intact. The vagina may have greater ligamentous support when the cervix is retained and therefore may be less likely to *prolapse*, or stretch out. At least one study has shown an increased incidence of prolapse within ten years in 60 percent of women who underwent total hysterectomy.

Doctors in London recently completed an excellent study comparing supracervical and total hysterectomy. In the largest study of this topic to date, published in the *New England Journal of Medicine*, these researchers did not find a significant difference in sexual enjoyment between women who had supracervical and those who had total hysterectomy. They did, however, find that supracervical hysterectomy caused significantly fewer surgical complications, took less time to do, and resulted in women leaving the hospital sooner. Since the study ran for only 12 months, they could not determine whether supracervical hysterectomy improved the risk of prolapse or not. This study provides the strongest support to date for replacing many total hysterectomies with supracervical hysterectomies—a shorter, safer procedure is a good choice, even if the outcomes from both types of surgery are similar.

Removing the cervix at the time of hysterectomy became standard after doctors realized that doing so could prevent cervical cancer. Cervical cancer was once considered unstoppable, but Pap smears have dramatically reduced the risk of this cancer. Cervical cancers develop very slowly, and having a regular Pap smear can reveal cervical abnormalities in plenty of time to treat them without hysterectomy. Women with a history of abnormal Pap smears may want to seriously consider having their cervix removed at the time of hysterectomy since these women are at higher risk of cancer.

QUALITY OF LIFE

More than two-thirds of all women who have hysterectomies say they are satisfied with the results. About a third express regret or have troublesome side effects they had not anticipated. Perhaps the most extensive study on this topic, the Maine Women's Health Study, surveyed more than four hundred women after hysterectomy for fibroids and found marked improvement in pain, fatigue, bleeding, and sexual dysfunction. Most women reported better mental and physical health and an improved quality of life after hysterectomy. However, pelvic pain persisted in 5 percent of women, and problems with urination persisted in 9 percent. In addition, new symptoms such as hot flashes appeared in 13 percent of women, weight gain in 12 percent, depression in 8 percent and lack of interest in sex appeared in 7 percent of respondents (some women had several symptoms, so adding these percentages together overestimates the number of women with problems).

Hysterectomies are frequently performed on women who are at an age when they may be under many other life stresses. Working women (in or out of the home), women with ill parents, women under financial stress, or women feeling pressured by their multiple roles may experience problems with fibroids as an additional stressor. In this context, removing the uterus can potentially add to physical problems and stress, triggering depression and diminishing quality of life. More commonly, treating fibroids with surgery will increase stress only until after recovery, at which point improved health will make dealing with other stressors easier.

Sex after Hysterectomy

Sexual function may be either helped or hindered by a hysterectomy. Most studies show that sex is better after the hysterectomy since the fibroids and their symptoms have disappeared. This is particularly true if bleeding, pressure, and pain were hampering your sex life before surgery. If you suffer complications from surgery, however, your sex life could be made worse. In rare cases, pelvic pain can be a side effect of hysterectomy, making sex painful or impossible.

If your sex life is good before hysterectomy, it is generally likely to remain so afterward. Women who have a greater orgasmic response before hysterectomy are the most likely to report improved sexual function after hysterectomy, according to a 1997 study in the *British Journal of Obstetrics and Gynaecology*. The same study reported that women who have unsatisfactory sexual relations before surgery, poor knowledge of reproductive anatomy, and negative expectations for surgery are more likely to have worse sex lives after hysterectomy.

Although most studies have concluded that women engage in more *frequent* sex after hysterectomy, the issue of *quality* of the sexual experience has not been fully addressed. Several studies have shown that an abdominal hysterectomy has no adverse effect on sexual function, provided the vagina is not shortened excessively and that the ovaries are not removed. Other studies have reported decreased libido, psychological complications, or problems with intercourse after hysterectomy.

Sexual Expression

Many women's feelings of sexual identity, sexual attractiveness, and even their completeness as people are expressed in sex. Sex is a physical, emotional, psychological, and social event. As you become aroused, this activates the skin, sexual organs, and nerves. Muscular tension and blood flow to the genital area increase, ultimately resulting in orgasm—short, intense, rhythmic muscular contractions that pleasantly release muscular and nervous tension built up in the vagina, perineum, anus, and all over the body. Most women experience orgasm primarily through stimulation of the clitoris, although for some women orgasm involves the uterus and cervix as well.

The vagina, the uterus, the ovaries, and the cervix all sing a song in the chorus of sexual pleasure. A rush of blood into the pelvic region helps prepare the body for sex. The vagina dilates and expands prior to intercourse; the uterus also expands during sexual arousal. Sexual pleasure may also be enhanced by the nerve supply to the pelvic organs; these nerves intimately surround the cervix and link it to both the bladder and the upper vagina. In studies of sexual function, approximately 15 percent of women report a sensation of strong uterine contractions during orgasm. The ovaries make about half of the body's testosterone (yes, women do have testosterone, although men produce much more). According to some studies of sexual function, testosterone increases the sensitivity of the external genitals, increases a women's openness to psychosexual stimulation, and creates sex that is more gratifying. This harmony of organs is another strong reason for not reflexively removing normal ovaries or a normal cervix at the time of surgery for fibroids.

Complications and Side Effects

Hysterectomy is major surgery and as such is potentially life threatening. For premenopausal women without cancer, most studies estimate that about one in a thousand will die from a hysterectomy. Most deaths are from blood clots developing in the legs and traveling to the lungs, or from infections that cannot be controlled. Obese women and women in poor health are at higher risk of dying during or shortly after surgery. Of course, this small risk of death must be weighed against the similarly small risk of dying from uncontrolled bleeding due to fibroids or against the daily pain of living with debilitating symptoms.

Altogether, about one in ten women has some mild, short-term complications from hysterectomy. As many as 3 percent of women who have hysterectomies may develop urinary tract infections. Since the bladder is dissected away from the uterus during hysterectomy, it can also be bruised, cut, or damaged in the process. Internal organs or blood vessels are sometimes accidentally injured, and this can necessitate additional surgery to repair the damage. Hernias; damage to the ureters, vaginal, or fallopian tubes; prolapse; and pelvic pain are rare complications (happening in approximately one in a hundred surgeries). Blood transfusions are also necessary in about one of every ten hysterectomies. These risks are similar to those associated with myomectomy.

A woman who has had a hysterectomy will tend to enter menopause an average of five years earlier than a woman with a uterus. Even if they are not removed, the ovaries age rapidly after hysterectomy because surgery reduces the ovaries' blood supply.

An estimated 20 percent of women have some short-term sexual dysfunction after hysterectomies, and this number more than doubles if the ovaries are also removed. Depression after hysterectomy (and other major surgery) is common, but usually does not last long.

Hysterectomy is a difficult surgery, but it's generally safe. Of the invasive therapies, hysterectomy is a good choice for some women with fibroids. Women who want all of their fibroids gone once and for all, and who don't want more children, are the best candidates. Simultaneous removal of the cervix or ovaries is frequently recommended, but this is usually not necessary unless you have a history of abnormal Pap smears or a family history of ovarian cancer. Both quality of life and sexual function are usually (but not always) improved by a hysterectomy. Although hysterectomy is currently the most common invasive treatment for women with fibroids, it's much more than many women need, so be sure you have considered all of the less invasive options before choosing this procedure.

BEFORE SURGERY

You can prepare for surgery by eating well, exercising, and making sure that you are in good overall physical shape before surgery. Building up your strength and stamina increases the chances that the surgery will go well and makes for a shorter recovery time. Because surgery is physically and emotionally stressful, you should bring relaxation tapes or tapes of your favorite music with you to the hospital (you can even ask to hear the tapes during surgery). Anything that buoys your mental attitude and relieves stress will probably help your recovery.

AFTER SURGERY

It can take months to recover completely from surgery. After abdominal myomectomy or abdominal hysterectomy, you will be in the hospital for two to three days. The first twenty-four hours are usually the worst. Although you will be receiving strong medicine to help relieve your pain, it is not always possible to control postoperative pain quickly. Sometimes several dosage changes are needed, and this means you may be in pain right after surgery.

The first day after surgery will probably be spent in bed. You may be asked to get up and dangle your legs at the side of the bed or perhaps sit in a chair. Even though you don't feel well, it's a good idea to do these things. One possible complication of surgery is the formation of blood clots in the legs; getting out of bed can reduce the risk of these clots. Right after surgery you will probably have a catheter draining urine from your bladder. During surgery this catheter is used to monitor the amount of urine that your body produces. Immediately after surgery it keeps you from having to get up and go to the bathroom at a time when it would probably be too painful to do so. Once the catheter is no longer needed, usually after about twenty-four hours, it should be removed. The longer the catheter remains in place, the higher is the risk of getting a bladder infection from it. You probably will not eat anything on the first day after surgery, but an IV will provide all the fluids your body needs. If you do eat, take it slowly. If you feel nauseous, stop eating.

On the second day after surgery you will probably be moving around more and walking up and down the halls. You may also begin to take some food by mouth. Sometimes doctors will have you try liquids before giving you solid food. Once you can take solid food, your pain medication will probably be given by mouth instead of IV. Make no mistake: You can still get enough pain medication by mouth to control your pain. The pain medicine you're getting in the pills is not very different from that given in the IV; it's just that oral medications may not be very well absorbed right after surgery. When changing from IV to oral medication, you need to make sure your pain is still well controlled.

Some people try not to use pain medication under the theory that they'll "save it for when they really need it." This is a big mistake. Pain is much easier to fix when it's less severe. If you take two pain pills before your pain gets bad, it might prevent you from needing four pills later. Addiction to pain medication taken to relieve pain is very unusual. Study after study has shown that people who take pain medication appropriately after surgery, even strong medication such as morphine, do not become addicts. Don't make your postoperative course worse than it has to be: Take your medicine.

By the third day after surgery you should be walking around, eating regular food, urinating on your own. You may not have a bowel movement before you leave the hospital since some of the medications that you're taking can make you constipated. Doctors usually take passing gas as a sign of normal intestinal function after surgery.

Although you'll probably go home from the hospital around the third day, your recovery will take a bit longer. The first few days home from the hospital are usually difficult. In the hospital, there is very little you can do, so you're forced to rest. Once at home, the temptation just to "straighten up a little bit" or to make yourself dinner can be very strong. Try to resist this, at least for the first few days. While you're not likely to do any permanent damage from increasing your activity too quickly, it can put you in a fair amount of pain that will require more medication and more time to get under control.

The first two weeks after the hospital stay are a period of slow recovery. During this time you can expect to be taking pain medication around the clock. You also will have fairly limited ability to do normal activities. By the end of these two weeks you'll probably be walking around, dressing yourself, and possibly making your own meals. You may be able to do a few things outside of the house, but not much.

Over the next month, your activities will probably return to a normal level. Most people who work from home find themselves doing more and more work during this month. Those who work in an office rarely feel well enough to go back to the office until six weeks after surgery.

When the six-week postoperative recovery period is over, you might feel close to normal. You probably won't be using pain medication, and your activity level will be reasonably normal. One thing that many women notice after surgery is that they still feel fatigued long after most of the other symptoms are gone. This seems to be the effect of the body putting most of its energy toward healing. For up to two to three months (and sometimes longer) after surgery, many women still need to take naps, sleep longer at night, and just don't have their usual energy. Not everyone experiences this prolonged period of fatigue, but if you do experience it, remember that it's a normal part of recovery. Women who are physically fit before surgery seem to have less trouble with this kind of fatigue.

With regard to returning to exercise after surgery, the best advice is to proceed slowly and gradually. Walking is the best form of exercise to start after surgery. You can begin by walking just around your house, then around the block. Once these walks become easy, you can lengthen them. It's always better to stop before you're in pain than it is to push yourself. If you're able to walk two blocks one day without pain, the next day try three blocks. Don't try to see how far you can walk before the pain starts: Remember, you still have to make it home! Exercises such as sit-ups and weight-lifting should probably not be restarted for at least two months after surgery, and talk with your doctor about these things before you begin them.

HORMONE REPLACEMENT THERAPY

Most American women can expect to live a full third of their lives after menopause. For many women, entering into menopause brings relief from fibroid symptoms. After menopause, small fibroids usually stop causing problems.

Larger fibroids can stabilize or even shrink, possibly because the ovaries make significantly less estrogen than they made before menopause. However, menopause can bring its own set of symptoms. These symptoms appear suddenly in women entering into a surgically induced menopause. To control these symptoms, doctors often recommend replacing lost hormones with estrogen (and sometimes progestin) in pill form (called hormone replacement therapy or HRT).

Hormone replacement therapy has risks and benefits. About half the postmenopausal women in the United States take HRT; many are advised by their doctors to stay on HRT for life, not just to help with symptoms like hot flashes but also to reduce the risk of heart disease and osteoporosis. During menopause an estimated 75 percent of women experience hot flashes, vaginal dryness, and night sweats, and HRT relieves many of these symptoms. Despite early reports, HRT has no proven benefits in reducing heart attacks. In fact, in mid-2002, the Women's Health Initiative study of HRT was suddenly halted when it was determined that HRT use in study participants who still had a uterus showed increased risks of invasive breast cancer, coronary heart disease, stroke, and pulmonary embolisms.

Many women with fibroids are reluctant to begin hormone replacement therapy after menopause even if they have bothersome symptoms, worrying that HRT may prevent the natural shrinkage of fibroids. We have not found that giving HRT to women with fibroids who are experiencing menopausal symptoms and needing some form of short-term medical therapy for relief usually causes problems. It can sometimes cause irregular bleeding, but this is usually easy to manage with dosage changes.

How you take the hormones may make a difference in the

effect on fibroids. Susan Love, M.D., coauthor of *Dr. Susan Love's Hormone Book*, cited a yearlong randomized controlled trial conducted at Dr. Zekai Tahir Burak Women's Hospital in Ankara, Turkey. In this study women who received hormones through a skin patch had some fibroid growth, although none was seen when HRT was taken in pill form.

So-called "designer estrogens" or selective estrogen receptor moderators (SERMs) attempt to send estrogen to sites where it is needed, such as bones, heart, and blood vessels, and keep it away from the breasts and uterus, where problems such as cancer can occur. These drugs promise the benefits of HRT without the risk and may be good choices for some women (see chapter 10).

More studies are needed to assess the risks of HRT on women with fibroids. At this point, it is safe to say that some types of hormone therapy may cause fibroid growth, but each woman's experience is unique. For women with symptoms of menopause who need HRT, a trial period of six months followed by a pelvic exam and ultrasound is a prudent course of action. If fibroids continue to grow, or if symptoms get worse, the dose can be changed, or therapy can be discontinued and other treatments can be tried.

Chapter 14

Into the Future

Interesting new approaches to fibroid treatment are appearing on the horizon. These include preventive approaches and research into promising new drugs, new forms of surgery, alternative therapies, and even gene therapy. One day, these exciting new approaches will almost surely make current treatments obsolete. Hopefully, doctors in the future will laugh at the idea of anything as barbaric as cutting someone open to take out her fibroids!

NEW DRUGS

At the Center for Uterine Fibroids at Brigham and Women's Hospital in Boston, a major research center, several new drugs are being tested. One of the most promising is called pirfenidone. Pirfenidone (brand name Deskar) is an antifibrotic drug that inhibits collagen production and blocks growth factors known to affect fibroids. In test tubes this drug prevents fibroids from growing. Pirfenidone may not only shrink fibroids, but could even be used to prevent them. In current studies in Europe (it is not approved for use in the United States), pirfenidone is being taken in the form of a gelcap three times per day.

Another new drug being tested is tibilone, a hormone medication already used in Europe that appears to have some advantages over standard hormone therapy and may shrink fibroids. Tibilone is currently being tested for use in the United States.

As modest as it might seem, the development of animal research models for fibroids is an encouraging development. For many years scientists have had great difficulty finding any animal useful for research that can develop fibroids at all, which has slowed research. In a report published in 1995, however, a line of animals called the Eker rat, identified at the M. D. Anderson Cancer Center at the University of Texas, was identified. The Eker rat can spontaneously develop muscular tumors similar to uterine fibroids. In early experiments, estrogen makes these tumors grow, and depriving them of estrogen or giving antiestrogen drugs such as tamoxifen makes them shrink. Animal studies are important in testing drugs before trying them on humans. The Eker rat should help shorten the time it takes to bring new drugs and other treatments for fibroids and provide scientists insight into the development of fibroids.

NEW FORMS OF INVASIVE THERAPY

During the last decade, a wide range of new invasive options have been introduced. Some have shown tremendous promise over the last few years, but do need further study.

Uterine Fibroid Embolization

Uterine fibroid embolization continues to be refined. Currently, the procedure uses materials that permanently block uterine arteries. However, a few investigators are experimenting with a temporary form of embolization using only the gelatin sponge, which can dissolve. This form of embolization has shown some good results in preliminary studies and may have long-term benefits for certain women, such as those who want children.

Endometrial Ablation

If you are a candidate for a hysteroscopic procedure, and bleeding is the main problem you are having from your fibroids, you should at least discuss with your doctor the idea of endometrial ablation. During an endometrial ablation, the entire lining of the uterus is burned or removed using a type of wire loop. Because the endometrium is the area from which menstrual bleeding occurs, if the endometrium is burned away completely, there will be no more menstrual bleeding. That's right, no more periods. This is a procedure reserved for women who do not want to have children. Clearly, the elimination of the endometrial lining would interfere with the ability of a fertilized egg to attach to the uterine lining.

Endometrial ablation has been in use for over twenty years and some experts estimate that it could replace as many as 20 percent of the hysterectomies that are performed in the United States. Very carefully done studies of endometrial ablation show very high satisfaction rates among women who have had this procedure to control their bleeding, but most of these studies did not include women who had uterine fibroids since fibroids can distort the uterus and make the procedure harder to perform. Early equipment and technique made this a treatment not generally recommended for women with fibroids, as it generally required an evenly shaped endometrial lining to be carried out safely, and fibroids often distort the endometrium. However, time and advances in technology are changing this recommendation, and with new equipment and further study, endometrial ablation may have a place in the menu of treatment options for uterine fibroids.

If you have several small submucosal fibroids, and these can be removed with hysteroscopy, then there is good reason to believe that endometrial ablation would further improve the chance that your bleeding will be permanently cured. If your fibroids are large, or not submucosal, endometrial ablation might still help with heavy bleeding, but the odds of success are unknown simply because the procedure hasn't been well studied in women with nonsubmucosal fibroids.

Because the entire endometrium is burned away, this is not a good procedure if you want to retain your fertility. Strangely, even though a normal pregnancy can't be supported, it still may be possible to have an early pregnancy after endometrial ablation; therefore, the use of birth control after the procedure is recommended.

Myoma Coagulation (Myolysis)

Myolysis, a technique for destroying uterine fibroids without removing them, has been around since the late 1980s. The procedure was introduced in Europe and subsequently introduced in the United States in 1992. The technique has very vocal advocates but has not become widely accepted.

Myolysis is a laparoscopic procedure, and so it requires no

overnight hospital stay and has a much shorter recovery period than open surgical procedures. The original technique was to burn the myomas with a laser fiber inserted into the body of the fibroid. Subsequent modifications of this technique have substituted electrically charged needles, heated needles, and freezing cold probes inserted into the fibroids. The principle of all of these techniques is the same. Energy (whether in the form of laser, electricity, cold, or heat) damages the myoma blood vessels, causing the fibroid to subsequently die. Because the probes are inserted into the uterus under direct vision, they can be carefully placed only where there is abnormal fibroid tissue.

Although there was initially great interest in these techniques, they have not become widely accepted because of some significant problems. First, in studies in which the uterus was examined weeks to months after the procedure, between 50 and 100 percent of patients had thick scars forming between the uterus and the intestines. These scars are potentially a source of chronic pain and could possibly interfere with pregnancy.

Also, in a case series of three women who got pregnant shortly after myolysis, two had rupture of the uterus during their pregnancy. In one of these women, the baby died. For these reasons, myolysis has generally not been recommended to any woman who wishes to get pregnant in the future.

Well-designed studies of myolysis comparing this procedure to more standard techniques, such as myomectomy, are seriously lacking. The published studies are generally of poor quality and do not provide enough information on complications and recurrence risks for this procedure to be recommended for general use.

A recent study suggested that combining myolysis with endometrial ablation would improve bleeding and reduce recurrence rates more than performing either of these procedures alone. However, in this study, four out of fifty-two patients had serious complications. This high complication rate is much greater than that seen with more accepted techniques.

So far, the technique of myoma control using myolysis can only be considered experimental. As with any new treatment lacking in comprehensive research and clinical data, until better information on the safety and long-term success rates of this technique are available, we cannot recommend it.

High-Intensity Focused Ultrasound (HIFUS)

Although this procedure may sound like something out of a science fiction novel, it is already possible to vaporize fibroids without invasive techniques using focused ultrasound energy. Researchers in Boston are experimenting with a new high-intensity focused ultrasound (HIFUS) technique that focuses several ultrasound beams on a single fibroid. Guided by an MRI, HIFUS can coagulate a fibroid without requiring any cuts on the body. Although regular ultrasound is harmless, focused ultrasound causes tissue to vibrate, heating it until cells die. HIFUS is quite slow at the moment; it can take two hours to vaporize a small one- to two-centimeter fibroid. However, this technology will surely get faster and better and may soon help many women with fibroids and perhaps other tumors, including breast cancer.

In the first pilot study of this new technique, conducted at Harvard Medical School, fibroids were "melted away" by the new procedure in nine women who each had one to five fibroids. The women were treated for four hours at a time, and the results were confirmed by pathological reports, according to the lead researcher in the study, Dr. Clare Tempany. Because it takes so long and is so expensive, the treatment is not a practical alternative, but one day may well be.

Gamma Knife

The gamma knife is another new technique with potential applications to fibroids. The gamma knife is used now for very delicate brain surgery. It can accurately target and destroy small tumors in the most sensitive area of the body. A huge machine weighing eighteen tons, the gamma knife uses 201 beams of highly focused gamma rays, with these beams of ionizing radiation intersecting with an accuracy of less than one-tenth of a millimeter. The gamma knife can precisely destroy one small area without significant damage to surrounding tissues. Patients can go home in about half a day from a one-treatment, outpatient procedure. There are no reports of gamma knife treatments of fibroids, but this may be a direction for future research. Other minimally invasive techniques such as radio frequency ablation, which uses radio waves to destroy tumors, may find their way into use for treating fibroids.

ALTERNATIVE THERAPY

Herbal medicine, homeopathy, and acupuncture are among the alternative therapies women sometimes try for fibroids. Better research on these and many other alternative therapies is desperately needed before doctors can recommend them. Luckily, more research on some alternative therapies is underway, funded by the federal government through the National Center for Complementary and Alternative Medicine in Silver Spring, Maryland. Already, Columbia University in New York has begun a research project on traditional Chinese herbal formulas for fibroids.

GENETICS

The completion of the Human Genome Project has given us a great deal of insight into the mystery of the human body and the forty-six human chromosomes that contain the blueprints for the entire body. Gene therapy on humans formally began in September of 1990, when two girls with a rare congenital immune deficiency were injected with experimentally "corrected" T cells from their own bodies. The girls showed improved immune function that allowed them to continue with their lives.

Although gene therapy is highly experimental at the moment, it may someday help women who suffer from fibroids. Briefly, gene therapy involves the transfer of certain genes from the test tube into a patient's body, triggering a therapeutic benefit. Recombinant DNA technology, involving minute transfers of material at the molecular level, may make possible developments even science fiction writers cannot imagine.

Three basic strategies that could theoretically be adapted to the treatment of fibroids are (1) therapy to correct the genetic defects that cause fibroids; (2) stimulating the immune system to attack fibroid cells; and (3) cytotoxic therapy, which could directly destroy abnormal cells such as those that multiply into fibroids. According to researchers at the University of Michigan in Ann Arbor, cytotoxic gene therapy at this moment looks to be the most promising of the three in the future treatment of fibroids.

Scientists in Boston, too, are looking at two particular genes that may play some future role in treating fibroids. Researchers have zeroed in on chromosomes 6, 7, 12, and 14, and mutations in two particular genes called the HMGIC and HMGIY genes. These genes have an indirect role in cell growth; in the future, they may prove to be one of the keys to controlling fibroids. "As the effects of genes, including HMGIC and HMGIY, are determined, new treatments to prevent leiomyoma formation or growth may be developed," Harvard University researcher E. A. Stewart stated. "As we gain understanding of the molecular events that cause benign gynecologic conditions, such as leiomyomas, safer and more effective treatments might be found as we enter the 2lst century."

FINAL THOUGHT

Even with all of these exciting developments on the horizon, a magic pill that makes fibroids disappear without side effects will probably not be found in our lifetimes. Nevertheless, good medical treatments are available now. Learn about fibroids, make your treatment choices with the help of your medical doctor, and get back to enjoying life.

Continue to educate yourself not only about fibroids, but also about good health. Choose good health behaviors. Eating nutritiously and exercising several times a week will help you live a longer and healthier life with or without fibroids. Go in for medical checkups as recommended. Avoid whatever stresses you can and don't obsessively ruminate about your fibroids. Above all else, remember that you are not your disease. A sound body and mind, a healthy love of life, and continuing optimism and hope will help you move confidently through medical treatment and into the future.

Glossary

Abdominal myomectomy: An operation to remove uterine fibroids done through an incision in the abdomen. The most common type of myomectomy.

Ablation: To remove or excise tissue. Often used to describe the burning or coagulation of the endometrial lining to prevent excessive bleeding.

Acupuncture: Many thousand-year-old technique for treating illness by inserting very thin needles into various points in the body.

Adenomyosis: A condition in which endometrial tissue that usually lines the uterus grows backward into the deep muscle outside the uterine lining. Sometimes associated with pain, enlargement of the uterus, and bleeding. Can be confused with uterine fibroids on physical examination and sometimes ultrasound.

Adhesion: A type of scar tissue that often forms inside the body after surgery. Most adhesions do not cause any problems, but they may occasionally cause pelvic pain.

Adrenaline: A stress hormone produced by the adrenal gland located near the kidney. This hormone is involved in the "flight or fight" response to stress.

Amenorrhea: The absence of menstruation. "Primary amenorrhea" means that menstruation has never begun. This term is used to describe a woman who has otherwise reached the age at which she should be menstruating but has not yet started. "Secondary amenorrhea" means that periods have once occurred but have since stopped for more than six months.

American College of Obstetrics and Gynecologists: The leading professional medical organization for gynecologists in the United States.

Anastomosis: A place where two hollow structures join together. Two blood vessels are said to anastomose if they meet and blood can flow one to the other.

Anemia: A condition in which the number of circulating red blood cells is reduced, usually a symptom of other disease. Red blood cells carry oxygen and are crucial for normal functioning of bodily organs.

Angiography: A technique for injecting dye into the blood vessels. The dye can then be seen using X rays or other techniques, allowing mapping of the course of blood vessels.

Anovulation (anovulatory): Refers to a menstrual cycle during which no egg is released from the ovary. Typically, the egg is released from an ovarian cyst halfway through the menstrual cycle. It is the release of the egg and the subsequent drop in progesterone levels that bring on a predictable period. In the absence of ovulation, menses can become irregular and unpredictable.

Autologous blood donation: The donation of a person's own blood prior to surgery, to be used in case a transfusion is necessary. The donated blood can be stored for up to thirty days before it must be used or discarded.

Averse (as in "surgery averse"): Disliking or being disinclined to do something.

Benign tumor: *Tumor* is a Latin word meaning "growth" and *be-*

nign means "noncancerous." A growth in the body, such as a fibroid, which is not cancerous.

Bimanual examination: A method of examining the uterus and ovaries. The doctor places two fingers into the vagina and one hand on the abdomen to feel these pelvic organs.

Biofeedback: A mind/body therapy that allows someone to monitor and modify physical functions, such as skin temperature, heart rate, or blood pressure.

Biopsy: Removing a small amount of tissue in order to test it usually to determine whether it is benign or malignant.

Calcified: Filled with calcium deposits. These calcium deposits make structures both easier to see on ultrasound or X ray and firmer to the touch.

Catheter: A hollow tube. A urinary catheter inserted into the bladder drains urine out of the body.

Centimeter: A metric measurement of length. There are two and a half centimeters in one inch.

Cervix: The lower portion of the uterus. The cervix is the entrance to the uterus through which menstrual blood passes out into the vagina and through which sperm must pass in order to cause a pregnancy. The cervix is usually about one to two inches long and narrower than the rest of the uterus. The vagina connects to the uterus at the cervix.

Collateral blood flow: Blood flow from other sources. If there is good collateral flow to an organ, then removing some of the blood supply will not injure that organ.

Complete blood count: A blood test that measures the number and type of red and white blood cells in circulation. It can reveal the presence of anemia.

Computerized tomography (CAT or CT) scan: A procedure that takes cross-sectional images of internal organs to detect abnormalities that may not appear on a regular X ray. A technique for looking inside the body using X rays.

Corticosteroid: A type of hormone produced in the adrenal glands (small glands that sit on top of the kidneys). Synthetic corticosteroids are used to reduce inflammation and can be taken in pill form or used topically. There are many steroid hormones in the body, and they all have similarities in their basic structure but perform different functions.

Cortisol: Also called hydrocortisone. A steroid hormone produced by the adrenal gland.

Cryomyolysis: A technique for treating uterine fibroids that involves inserting a cold needle or fiber into the fibroid and freezing the blood supply.

Cryosurgery: *Cryo* means "cold," and cryosurgery uses freezing cold devices to kill or remove particular cells. Cryosurgery is used frequently in dermatology to remove skin lesions and is also used in gynecology to remove abnormal cells from the cervix. It has recently been introduced as a way to destroy uterine fibroids.

CT scan (computerized): A technique for looking inside the body using X rays.

Cyst: A fluid-filled sac. Cysts are very common throughout the body and in particular on the ovaries. A normal ovary in a menstruating woman produces cysts constantly. One cyst becomes larger each month, and it is this cyst that eventually releases an egg. The finding of cysts on an ultrasound in a woman who is still having periods is a normal finding.

Degeneration: Breaking down. A term used to describe shrinkage of fibroids that may occur when the fibroids do not get enough blood to sustain them.

Dysfunction: Abnormal functioning, impaired functioning, or inadequate functioning of an organ or part of the body.

Dysmenorrhea: Painful periods.

Dyspareunia: Pain during sexual intercourse. This pain is usually experienced at the entrance to the vagina (called the "introitus") or deep inside the vagina. Dyspareunia can result from skin irritation, muscular spasm, nerve problems, or unknown reasons.

Dysplasia: An abnormal development of tissue. Cervical dysplasia is the presence of abnormal—often precancerous—cells on the cervix.

EKG: Electrocardiogram. A technique for examining the electrical activity of the heart.

Endogenous: Something the body creates rather than something given from outside. For example, the adrenal glands produce endogenous steroid hormones, but these drugs can also be given exogenously (or in pill form).

Endometrial ablation: A procedure in which the lining of the uterus is destroyed, usually by burning. This technique can reduce bleeding very successfully. It is generally used only in the absence of significant uterine fibroids.

Endometrial biopsy: A method of taking a small sample of cells from the endometrial lining or inside of the uterus. This technique is most often used to rule out endometrial cancer as a cause of abnormal vaginal bleeding. It has largely replaced the D&C (dilatation and curettage) as a means of finding uterine cancer. It is done in a doctor's office, usually without sedation or anesthesia, and can cause menstrual cramps.

Endometrial hyperplasia: See Hyperplasia.

Endometrial lining: The thin, innermost portion of the uterus. A fertilized egg implants in the endometrial lining to begin its development. A portion of this lining is lost every month with a menstrual period and regrows during the rest of the cycle.

Endometriosis: The cells that normally line the uterus may be found in other parts of the body. These cells can somehow migrate to the outside surface of the uterus, the ovaries, or other places in the pelvis. When this happens, the resulting condition is called endometriosis. These endometrial cells located outside the uterus can sometimes bleed and bring on irritation-causing pain. Endometriosis may be difficult to diagnose and is best diagnosed with laparoscopy and biopsies of areas that are suspicious.

Endometrium: The thin lining of the inside of the uterus. It is the sloughing or falling off of this endometrial lining that produces menstrual bleeding. More than half of the "blood" in menstrual bleeding actually consists of endometrial cells.

Endorphins: A group of naturally occurring substances that are produced in the brain and reduce pain.

Endoscopy: *Endo* means "inside," and scope is a viewing device. Endoscopy uses thin telescopes attached to cameras or eyepieces to allow doctors to see inside various parts of the body. Colonoscopy, in which a camera is inserted into the rectum to look at the colon, is a form of endoscopy. Laparoscopy, in which a camera is inserted through an incision in the belly button to look in the pelvis or abdomen, is also endoscopy. Hysteroscopy, in which a camera is similarly inserted through the cervix to look inside the uterus, is a third type of endoscopy.

Estriol: A weak form of estrogen.

Estrogen: Refers to a group of sex hormones that play a major role in the menstrual cycle and are partially responsible for the development of female sexual characteristics. Estrogen is produced in the ovaries, fat cells, and skin. There are three main forms of estrogen: estrone, estradiol, and estriol.

Fallopian tubes: The two thin tubes that link the ovaries and the uterus. The sperm and egg generally unite in the fallopian tubes to create a fertilized embryo.

Fascia, fascial layer: A thick tissue layer that acts as a structural support in the body.

Femoral artery: A large blood vessel that supplies the lower extremity.

Fibroid: A common term for a myoma, a benign muscular tumor of the uterus.

Fluoroscope: A device for examining the body with X rays.

Follicle-stimulating hormone (FSH): A female hormone produced in the pituitary gland that has a role in the menstrual cycle, helping the egg to mature.

Gastrointestinal: Relating to the stomach, intestines, or digestive system.

Gelatin sponge pledgets: Small foam particles that are used to temporarily block blood vessels.

Gene therapy: An emerging medical treatment using information about the role of particular genes in the treatment of disease. Gene therapy aims to improve the function of abnormal body parts by changing the basic instructions (the genes) present in every cell.

GnRH agonists: A class of drugs that temporarily shrink fibroids in most women. These drugs act like gonadotropin-releasing hormone (GnRH), a hormone produced in the brain that stimulates production of FSH and LH.

Gram: A metric measurement of weight or mass. There are twenty-eight grams in an ounce. A milligram is one-thousandth of a gram.

Hemorrhage: Uncontrolled bleeding.

Hormone: A class of chemicals secreted in an organ or gland that stimulate activity somewhere else in the body, or that trigger the secretion of another hormone.

Hormone replacement therapy (HRT): Taking hormones such as estrogen and progesterone in an attempt to replace natural hormones no longer produced by the body.

Hypermenorrhea: A medical term used to describe an increase in menstrual bleeding whether at the time of the expected period or between periods.

Hyperplasia: Excessive growth of normal cells in an organ. Endometrial hyperplasia occurs when the endometrial cells divide more rapidly than normal, but the individual cells are still normal in appearance. That is, the cells do not become dysplastic or malignant.

Hypothalamus: An organ in the brain that produces hormones.

Hysterectomy: Surgical removal of the uterus. The term *hysterec-*

tomy, even when described as a "total hysterectomy," does not mean removal of the ovaries.

Hysteroscope: A system using cameras to see inside the uterine cavity. The camera is inserted through the cervix.

Incontinence: Involuntary loss of urine or feces. Urinary incontinence is a very common and troubling condition that is under-diagnosed and undertreated.

Inflammation: Irritation.

Interventional radiologist: A radiologist with advanced training in using minimally invasive techniques to diagnose and treat disease.

Intramural fibroids: Uterine fibroids found within the muscle wall of the uterus. These fibroids do not stick out above the surface of the uterus, nor do they protrude into the uterine cavity. They may be associated with abnormal bleeding or pain.

Intrauterine: Occurring inside the uterus.

Intravenous pyelogram (IVP): A medical test in which dye is injected into a vein. The dye collects in the urinary system, identifying blockages or abnormalities in the system.

Isthmus: The lower segment of the uterus, just above the cervix.

IUD: Intrauterine device. A small plastic or metal device inserted into the uterus, typically used for birth control. The IUD prevents pregnancy by interfering with normal fertilization (joining of sperm and egg).

Kegel exercises: Exercises to strengthen the muscles of the pelvic floor.

Keloid: A thick, overgrown scar.

Laparohysterectomy (or laparoscopic hysterectomy): The removal of the uterus through a small incision in the abdominal wall using a laparoscope.

Laparomyomectomy (or laparoscopic myomectomy): The removal of fibroids using a laparoscope.

Laparoscope: A hollow telescope that can be inserted through a small incision in the belly. This allows a doctor to see inside the abdomen and pelvis without needing to make a large incision.

Laser: Amplified focused light that emits heat at close range. Can be used to burn or vaporize tissue with limited blood loss.

Leiomyoma: Another name for fibroid, a benign tumor arising from the smooth muscle tissue of the uterus.

Leiomyosarcoma: A malignant tumor or cancer in the smooth muscles of the uterus that may be confused with fibroids on physical examination.

Libido: Sexual drive.

Luteinizing hormone (LH): A female hormone that plays a role in the monthly menstrual cycle, helping the developing egg or follicle to secrete progesterone that can help a fetus develop.

Malignancy or malignant tumor: A growth in the body that is cancerous. Cancerous tumors spread to other organs and can invade deeply into tissues.

Menometrorrhagia: Irregular and heavy bleeding that includes heavy bleeding at the time of the periods and bleeding that occurs more frequently than every twenty-one days, typically between normal periods.

Menopause: Technically, menopause means the last menstrual period. A woman after age forty who experiences no periods for longer than twelve months is generally considered to have had menopause. The term *climacteric* means the area or period of time around the menopause, a time that is commonly referred to as perimenopause. The average age of menopause in the United States is 51.4 years. Ninety-five percent of women will have menopause between the ages of forty and sixty.

Menorrhagia: From the Latin words for "menses" and "to burst forth." Menorrhagia describes heavy or extended menstrual flow. This is more precisely defined as having menstrual periods that last more than eight days or during which more than 80 cc of blood is lost.

Menses: Monthly bleeding episodes, typically occurring every twenty-one to thirty-five days. Menses usually last between four and seven days, and bleeding results in less than 80 cc a month of blood loss.

Metrorrhagia: Bleeding between periods or bleeding that occurs more frequently than every twenty-one days.

Microcatheters: Small hollow tubes used to introduce material into blood vessels.

Microspheres: Tiny plastic balls used to block off arteries during uterine artery embolization.

Morcellation: Cutting something into small pieces. The term is used in relation to laparoscopic procedures in which fibroids are cut into small bits that may be easily removed from the body without needing large incisions on the abdomen.

MRI/MRA: Magnetic resonance imaging or magnetic resonance angiography; an imaging process using magnetic energy that very accurately maps the interior of parts of the body.

Myolysis: A medical treatment that destroys muscular tissue, such as fibroids.

Myoma: Another name for fibroid.

Myomectomy: Surgery to remove fibroids from the uterus without removing the uterus. *Myoma* refers to the fibroid tumor and *ectomy* means "removal."

Myometrium: The muscular portion of the uterus. Distinct from the *serosa*, or outer covering of the uterus, and from the *endometrium*, or inner lining. Fibroids contained within the myometrium are called *intramural*.

Necrose, necrotic: Dead tissue.

Norethindrone: A synthetic progesterone-like hormone commonly used in birth control pills.

Oligomenorrhea: Infrequent menstrual periods. Usually refers to periods that happen less often than every thirty-five days.

Oophorectomy: Surgical removal of one or both ovaries. If both ovaries are removed, can also be referred to as castration.

Osteoporosis: Thinning of the bones. It is associated with an increased risk for fractures.

Ovarian cyst: See Cyst.

Ovaries: The sex glands in the female body. These glands are responsible for the monthly production of the egg, as well as estrogen and progesterone.

Pedunculated fibroid: A fibroid attached to the uterus by a narrow stalk that is usually easy to remove. These fibroids hang from the outside or inside of the uterus but may be less likely to cause problems when they are on the outside.

Perimenopausal: *Peri* means "around," so this term means "around the menopause." The technically correct term is *climacteric. Perimenopausal* is often used to describe women who are having some symptoms of decreasing ovarian function, such as hot flashes, but are still having periods.

Perineum: The portion of the body containing the opening to the vagina and rectum.

Phytoestrogens: Estrogen-like chemicals that are contained in plants. These chemicals generally have a mild estrogen-like activity if they are consumed. Soy products contain phytoestrogens.

Pitressin: A synthetic hormone that causes blood vessels to constrict or tighten. The natural version of this hormone helps regulate blood pressure. Also called vasopressin.

Pituitary: A structure in the brain that secretes hormones.

Polymenorrhea: Periods that are too frequent, meaning less than every twenty-one days apart.

Polyp: A small, fleshy protrusion. Polyps in the uterus and cervix are almost always benign (noncancerous).

Premenopausal: Technically means "before menopause" and so would refer to any woman who is still menstruating. Sometimes incorrectly used as an alternative term for perimenopausal.

Progesterone: A hormone made primarily in the ovaries. Progesterone supports developing pregnancy. The ovary produces progesterone after ovulation, and progesterone production drops if no fertilization of the egg occurs. The drop in progesterone is responsible for a typical monthly menstrual period.

Progestins: Synthetic variations of progesterone that tend to have similar effects to progesterone when taken in pill form.

Prognosis: A medical doctor's prediction of the course of a disease and an estimate of the chances of recovery.

Prolapse: The falling of an organ outside the body or outside of its normal location. Organs that may commonly prolapse in women are the vagina and uterus. The bladder can also prolapse, meaning that it can begin to fall through the vaginal canal and can eventually come out of the vaginal opening. This condition is more common in women who have had many children, are smokers, are obese, or who have chronic cough.

Prostaglandin: A hormone-like substance that can cause muscles to contract.

Pulmonary embolism (PE): A blood clot that travels to the lungs. This is a potentially deadly condition.

PVA: Polyvinyl alcohol. A form of plastic.

Rad: A measure of radiation dose.

Resectoscope: A medical instrument, like a hysteroscope, that can be used to remove tissue from inside the uterus. It uses a wire loop that conducts electrical energy. Can remove fibroids on the inner lining of the uterus, with the instrument entering through the cervix rather than through an incision.

Salpingo-oophorectomy: A surgical procedure that removes the ovaries and fallopian tubes.

Selective estrogen receptor modulator (SERM): A synthetic compound that acts like estrogen in some parts of the body and like other hormones in other body parts.

Semen analysis: Examination of sperm.

Serosa: A skinlike covering that lies over many internal organs. The outer layer of the uterus.

Sessile fibroid: A fibroid attached to the uterus with a broad stalk. A type of subserosal fibroid.

Side effect: An action or effect of a particular drug other than the one desired.

Slough: Fall off or fall out.

Steroid: A group of hormones all with similar chemical structure. Steroid hormones include estrogen, progesterone, and testosterone.

Submucosal fibroids: Fibroids that project into the cavity of the uterus, occupying or intruding on the space in which a fetus would develop.

Subserosal fibroids: Fibroids that are located just under the serosa or outermost layer of the uterus.

Synthetic steroid: A steroid hormone that is produced in the laboratory instead of the body.

Testosterone: A hormone in the steroid group. Testosterone is present in both men and women but in greater quantities in men. Testosterone plays an important role in male sexual development, and in sex drive in both men and women.

Tomography scan: A series of X-ray images coordinated by a computer to produce an image that looks like a slice taken through the body.

Ultrasound: High-frequency inaudible sound in the range of more than twenty thousand cycles per second, used for either diagnostic or therapeutic purposes. Ultrasound or ultrasonography distinguishes tissues that differ in density and elasticity, permitting a doctor or ultrasound technician to outline the shape of particular tissues or organs in the body.

Ureters: Small tubes that carry urine from the kidneys to the bladder.

Uterine artery embolization or uterine fibroid embolization: An invasive procedure in which the uterine arteries are blocked off, reducing the blood supply to the uterus to make fibroids shrink.

Uterus: The muscular female reproductive organ in which a fetus is carried.

Vagina: A muscular, membrane-covered tube that forms a passageway between the vulva and the cervix.

Vaginal hysterectomy: The removal of the uterus and cervix through the vagina, using surgical means.

Vascular: Having to do with the blood vessels of the body.

Vasopressin: A synthetic hormone that causes blood vessels to constrict or tighten. The natural version of this hormone helps regulate blood pressure. Also called Pitressin.

Vitamins: A group of organic substances found in foods or synthesized in the body that are essential for normal metabolism, growth, or development of the body.

White blood cells: Blood cells that act as part of the immune system, fighting infection.

Xenoestrogens: Steroid hormones that are chemically similar to estrogen but are not made in the body and do not derive from plants. *Xeno* means "foreign," so these hormones come from a "foreign source," meaning an animal other than a human.

X rays: High-energy electromagnetic waves that can penetrate most solid matter; used in diagnosis and therapy.

Bibliography

Chapter 1. Fibroids

Bernstein SJ, McGlynn EA, Siu AL, Roth CP, Sherwood MJ, Keesey JW, Kosecoff J, Hicks NR, Brook RH. "The appropriateness of hysterectomy. A comparison of care in seven health plans." Health Maintenance Organization Quality of Care Consortium. *JAMA* 1993 May 12;269 (18):2398-402.

Broder MS, et al. "The appropriateness of recommendations for hysterectomy." *Obstet Gynecol* 2000 Feb; 95(2):199-205.

D'esopo A. "Hysterectomy when the uterus is grossly normal." *Am J Obstet Gynecol* 1962 Jan:113-122.

Doyle JC. "Unnecessary hysterectomies: study of 6248 operations in thirty-five hospitals during 1948." *JAMA* 1953 Jan 31:360-365.

Faerstein E, Szklo M, Rosenshein N. "Risk factors for uterine leiomyoma: a practice-based case-control study. I. African-American heritage, reproductive history, body size, and smoking." *Am J Epidemiol* 2001 Jan 1;153(1):1-10.

Faerstein E, Szklo M, Rosenshein NB. "Risk factors for uterine leiomyoma: a practice-based case-control study. II. Atherogenic risk factors and potential sources of uterine irritation." *Am J Epidemiol* 2001 Jan 1;153(1):11-19.

Farquhar CM, Steiner CA. "Hysterectomy rates in the United States 1990-1997." *Obstet Gynecol* 2002 Feb;99(2):229-34.

Huneycutt HC, Davis JL. "All about hysterectomy." Reader's Digest Press, New York. c. 1977.

Kjerulff KH, Erickson BA, Langenberg PW. "Chronic gynecological conditions reported by US women: findings from the National Health Interview Survey, 1984 to 1992." *Am J Public Health* 1996 Feb;86(2): 195-9.

"Management of Uterine Fibroids." Evidence Report No. 34, AHRQ publication No. 01-E051. January 2001. Agency for Healthcare Research and Quality, Rockville, MD.

Marshall LM, Spiegelman D, Barbieri RL, Goldman MB, Manson JE, Colditz GA, Willett WC, Hunter DJ. "Variation in the incidence of uterine leiomyoma among premenopausal women by age and race." *Obstet Gynecol* 1997 Dec;90(6):967-73.

Miller NF. "Hysterectomy: therapeutic necessity or surgical racket?" *Am J Obstet Gynecol* 1945 Oct:804-10.

Parazzini F, et al. "Reproductive factors and risk of uterine fibroids." *Epidemiology* 1996 July;7(4):440-2.

Reiter RC, Gambone JC, Lench JB. "Appropriateness of hysterectomies performed for multiple preoperative indications." *Obstet Gynecol* 1992 Dec;80(6):902-5.

Samadi AR, Lee NC, Flanders WD, Boring JR 3rd, Parris EB. "Risk factors for self-reported uterine fibroids: a case-control study." *Am J Public Health* 1996 Jun;86(6):858-62.

Schwartz SM. "Epidemiology of uterine leiomyomata." *Clinical Obstetrics and Gynecology* 2001 June;44(2):316-26.

Chapter 2. What Are Fibroids?

Cancer Facts & Figures 2002. American Cancer Society. Georgia. 2002.

Kjerulff KH, Langenberg P., Seidman JD, Stolley PD, Guzinski GM. "Uterine leiomyomas. Racial differences in severity, symptoms and age at diagnosis." *J Reprod Med* 1996 Jul;41(7):483-90.

Ligon AH, Morton CC. "Genetics of uterine leiomyomata." *Genes Chromosomes Cancer* 2000 July;28(3):235-45.

Parker W, et al. "Uterine sarcomas in patients operated on for presumed leiomyoma and rapidly growing leiomyoma," *Obstet Gynecol* 1994 March;83(3):414-8.

The PDR Family Guide to Women's Health and Prescription Drugs. Medical Economics Data, New Jersey. 1994.

Stovall DW. "Clinical symptomatology of uterine leiomyomas," *Clinical Obstetrics and Gynecology* 2001 June;44(2):364-71.

Takamizawa S, Minakami H, Usui R, Noguchi S, Ohwada M, Suzuki M, Sato I. "Risk of complications and uterine malignancies in women undergoing hysterectomy for presumed benign leiomyomas." *Gynecol Obstet Invest* 1999;48(3):193-6.

Chapter 3. Diagnosing Fibroids

Bazot M, Cortez A, Darai E, Rouger J, Chopier J, Antoine JM, Uzan S. "Ultrasonography compared with magnetic resonance imaging for the diagnosis of adenomyosis: correlation with histopathology." *Hum Reprod* 2001 Nov;16(11):2427-33.

Bergholt T, Eriksen L, Berendt N, Jacobsen M, Hertz JB. "Prevalence and risk factors of adenomyosis at hysterectomy." *Hum Reprod* 2001 Nov;16(11):2418-21.

Chapter 4. Managing Symptoms

Berkeley AS, et al. "Abdominal myomectomy and subsequent fertility," *Surgery, Gynecology & Obstetrics* 1983 March;156(3):319-22.

Carlson KJ, Miller BA, Fowler FJ Jr. "The Maine Women's Health Study: I. Outcomes of hysterectomy." *Obstet Gynecol* 1994 Apr;83(4):556-65.

Carlson KJ, Miller BA, Fowler FJ Jr. "The Maine Women's Health Study: II. Outcomes of nonsurgical management of leiomyomas, abnormal bleeding, and chronic pelvic pain." *Obstet Gynecol* 1994 Apr;83(4):566-72.

Darling CA, Smith YA. "Understanding hysterectomies: sexual satisfaction and quality of life." *Journal of Sex Research* 1993 Nov;30(4):324-335.

Davis MA. "Sexuality and sexual dysfunction." *Journal of Psychology* 1998 Nov, v132.

Dennerstein L, et al. "Sexual response following hysterectomy and oophorectomy." *Obstet Gynecol* 1977 Jan;49(1):92-6.

Dubuisson JB, Chapron C, Fauconnier A, Babaki-Fard K. "Laparoscopic myomectomy fertility results." *Ann N Y Acad Sci* 2001 Sep;943:269-75.

Katz VL, et al. "Complications of uterine leiomyomas in pregnancy." *Obstet Gynecol* 1989 Apr;73(4):593-6.

Laumann EO, et al. "Sexual dysfunction in the United States: prevalence and predictors." *JAMA* 1999 Feb 10;281(6):537-44.

Nilsson L, Rybo G. "Treatment of menorrhagia." *Am J Obstet Gynecol* 1971 July 1;110(5):713-20.

Pritts EA. "Fibroids and infertility: a systematic review of the evidence." *Obstet Gynecol Surv* 2001 Aug;56(8):483-91.

Ubaldi F, Tournaye H, Camus M, Van der Pas H, Gepts E, Devroey P. "Fertility after hysteroscopic myomectomy." *Hum Reprod Update* 1995 Jan;1(1):81-90.

Verkauf BS. "Myomectomy for fertility enhancement and preservation," *Fertility & Sterility* 1992, July;58(1)1-15.

Chapter 5. Watchful Waiting

Basil JB, Horowitz IR. "Cervical carcinoma: contemporary management." *Obstet Gynecol Clin North Am* 2001 Dec;28(4):727-42.

Hulley S, Furberg C, Barrett-Connor E, Cauley J, Grady D, Haskell W, Knopp R, Lowery M, Satterfield S, Schrott H, Vittinghoff E, Hunninghake D. "Noncardiovascular disease outcomes during 6.8 years of hormone therapy: Heart and Estrogen/progestin Replacement Study follow-up (HERS II)." *JAMA* 2002 Jul 3;288(1):58-66.

Lass A. "Assessment of ovarian reserve—is there a role for ovarian biopsy?" *Hum Reprod* 2001 Jun;16(6):1055-7.

Newton KM, Buist DS, Keenan NL, Anderson LA, LaCroix AZ. "Use of alternative therapies for menopause symptoms: results of a population-based survey." *Obstet Gynecol* 2002 Jul;100(1):18-25.

Parker W, et al. "Uterine sarcomas in patients operated on for presumed leiomyoma and rapidly growing leiomyomà." *Obstetrics and Gynecology* 1994 March;83(3):414-8.

Reiter R, et al. "Routine hysterectomy for large asymptomatic uterine leioymyomata: a reappraisal." *Obstetrics and Gynecology* 1992 Apr;79(4):481-4.

Rymer J, Morris EP. Extracts from "Clinical evidence: Menopausal symptoms." *BMJ* 2000 Dec 16;321(7275):1516-9.

Schwartz PE. "Nongenetic screening of ovarian malignancies." *Obstet Gynecol Clin North Am* 2001 Dec;28(4):637-51.

Smith-Bindman R, Kerlikowske K, Feldstein VA, Subak L, Scheidler J, Segal M, Brand R, Grady D. "Endovaginal ultrasound to exclude endometrial cancer and other endometrial abnormalities." *JAMA* 1998 Nov 4;280(17):1510-7.

Chapter 6. Diet

Armstrong BK, et al. "Diet and reproduction hormones: A study of vegetarian and nonvegetarian postmenopausal women." *Journal of the National Cancer Institute* 1981 Oct;67(4):761-7.

Chiaffarino F, et al. "Diet and uterine myomas," *Obstetrics and Gynecology* 1999 Sept;94(3):385-8.

Diamond S. "Hormone pollution: synthetic estrogens and the cancer connection," *Alive Magazine: Canadian Journal of Health and Nutrition* Apr 30, 1997.

Franchinetti F, et al. "Oral magnesium successfully relieves premenstrual mood changes." *Gynecology* 1991 Aug;78(2):177-81.

Goldin BR, et al. "Estrogen excretion patterns and plasma levels in vegetarian and omnivorous women." *New England Journal of Medicine* 1982 December 16;307(25):1542-7.

Hu FB, Bronner L, Willett WC, Stampfer MJ, Rexrode KM, Albert CM, Hunter D, Manson JE. "Fish and omega-3 fatty acid intake and risk of coronary heart disease in women." *JAMA* 2002 Apr 10;287(14):1815-21.

Lithgow DM, Politizer WM. "Vitamin A in the treatment of menorrhagia," *South African Medical Journal* 1977 Feb 12;51(7):191-93.

London RS, et al. "The effect of alpha-tocopherol on premenstrual symptomatology: a double-blind study. II Endocrine correlates." *J Am Coll Nutr* 1984; 3(4):351-6.

Proctor ML, Murphy PA. "Herbal and dietary therapies for primary and secondary dysmenorrhoea (Cochrane Review)." In: Cochrane Library Issue 2, 2002. Oxford: Update Software.

Valtin H. "Drink at least eight glasses of water a day—Really? Is there scientific evidence for '8 x 8'?" *Am J Physiol Regu Physiol*, online 10.1152/ajpregu.00365.2002.

Weil A. "Ask Dr. Weil database—uterine fibroids, avoiding surgery for uterine fibroids." From the website www.drweil.com 3/2001.

Chapter 7. Exercise

Aganoff JA, Boyle GJ. "Aerobic exercise, mood states and menstrual cycle symptoms." *J Psychosom Res* 1994 Apr;38(3):183-92.

Choi PY, Salmon P. "Symptom changes across the menstrual cycle in competitive sportswomen, exercisers and sedentary women." *Br J Clin Psychol* 1995 Sept;34(Pt 3):447-60.

Frisch RE, et al. "Former athletes have a lower lifetime occurrence of breast cancer and cancers of the reproductive system." *Adv Exp Med Biol* 1992, 322:29-39.

Israel RG, et al. "Effects of aerobic training on primary dysmenorrhea symptomology in college females." *J Am Coll Health* 1985 June;33(6): 241-4.

Johnson WG, et al. "Macronutrient intake, eating habits, and exercise and moderators of menstrual distress in healthy women." *Psychosomatic Medicine* 1995 July-August;57(4):324-30.

Kaminski BT, Rzempoluch J. "Evaluation of the influence of certain epidemiologic factors on development of uterine myomas." *Wiad Lek* 1993 Aug;46(15-16):592-6.

Metheny WP, Smith RP. "The relationship among exercise, stress, and primary dysmenorrhea." *J Behav Med* 1989 Dec;12(6):569-86.

Prior JC, et al. "Conditioning exercise decreases premenstrual symptoms: a prospective, controlled 6-month trial." *Fertility & Sterility* 1987 March;47(3):402-8.

Steege JF, Blumenthal JA. "The effects of aerobic exercise on premenstrual symptoms in middle-aged women: a preliminary study." *J Psychosom Res* 1993, 37(2):127-33.

Chapter 8. Stress

Amodei N, et al. "Psychological treatments of dysmenorrhea: differential effectiveness for spasmodics and congestives." *J Behav Ther Exp Psychiatry* 1987 June;18(2):95-103.

Ballick L, et al. "Biofeedback treatment of dysmenorrhea." *Biofeedback and Self-Regulation* 1982 Dec;7(4):499-520.

Ben-Menachem M. "Treatment of dysmenorrhea: a relaxation therapy program." *Int. J Gynecol Obstet* 1980 Jan-Feb;17(4):340-2.

Brekhman GI. "Psychoemotional stress syndrome and uterine myoma." *Akush Ginekil (Mosk)* 1990 Feb;(2):13-17.

Brekhman GI. "Psycho-electoregulation in conservative treatment of patients with uterine myoma." *Akush Ginekol (Mosk)* 1991 Dec;(12):48-51.

Foksinski M, et al. "The level of typical biomarker of oxidative stress 8-hydroxy-2'-deoxyguanosine is higher in uterine myomas than in control tissues and correlates with the size of the tumor." *Free Radic Biol Med* 2000 Oct 1;29(7):597-601.

Kaminski BT, Rzempoluch J. "Evaluation of the influence of certain epidemiologic factors on development of uterine myomas." *Wiad Lek* 1993 Aug;46(15-16):592-6.

Loch EG, et al. "Treatment of premenstrual syndrome with a phytopharmaceutical formulation containing Vitex agnus castus." *Journal of Women's Health Gender Based Medicine* 2000 Apr;9(3):315-20.

Schwartz SM, Marshall LM, Baird DD. "Epidemiologic contributions to understanding the etiology of uterine leiomyomata." *Environ Health Perspect* 2000 Oct;108 Suppl 5:821-7.

Chapter 9. Alternative Medicine

Amato P, Christophe S., Mellon PL. "Estrogenic activity of herbs commonly used as remedies for menopausal symptoms." *Menopause* 2002 Mar-Apr;9(2):145-50.

Blumenthal M (ed). Expanded E Commission Monographs. Newton MA: Integrative Medicine Communications, 2000.

Brown DJ. "Vitex agnus castus Clinical Monograph." *Quarterly Review of Natural Medicine* Summer 1994.

DerMarderosian A (ed). *The Review of Natural Products*, Facts and Comparison, St. Louis Missouri. 1st ed. 2001.

Fletcher RH, Fairfield KM. "Vitamins for chronic disease prevention in adults: clinical applications." *JAMA* 2002 Jun 19;287(23):3127-9.

Helms JM. "Acupuncture for the management of primary dysmenorrhea." *Obstetrics and Gynecology* 1987 Jan;69(1):51-6.

Jones TK, Lawson BM. "Profound neonatal congestive heart failure caused by maternal consumption of blue cohosh herbal medication." *J Pediatrics* 1998;132:550-2.

Kotani N, et al. "Analgesic effect of a herbal medicine for treatment of primary dysmenorrhea—a double-blind study." *American Journal of Chinese Medicine* 1997, 25(2):205-12.

MacPherson H, Thomas K, Walters S, Fitter M. "The York acupuncture safety study: prospective survey of 34,000 treatments by traditional acupuncturists." *BMJ* 2001 Sep 1;323(7311):486-7.

Mehl-Madrona L. "Complementary medicine treatment of uterine fibroids: a pilot study." *Altern Ther Health Med* 2002 Mar-Apr;8(2):34-6.

Newton KM, Buist DS, Keenan NL, Anderson LA, LaCroix AZ. "Use of alternative therapies for menopause symptoms: results of a population-based survey." *Obstet Gynecol* 2002 Jul;100(1):18-25.

Proctor ML, Smith CA, Farquhar CM, Stones RW. "Transcutaneous electrical nerve stimulation and acupuncture for primary dysmenorrhoea *Cochrane Database Syst Rev* 2002; (1): CD002123.

Rein MS, Barbieri RL, Friedman AJ. "Progesterone: a critical role in the pathogenesis of uterine myomas." *Am J Obstet Gynecol* 1995 Jan;172(1 Pt 1):14-8.

Steinberger A. "The treatment of dysmenorrhea by acupuncture." *American Journal of Chinese Medicine* Spring 1981, 9(1):57-60.

Tanaka T. "Effects of herbal medicines on menopausal symptoms induced by gonadotropin-releasing hormone agonist therapy." *Clin Exp Obstet Gynecol* 2001;28(1):20-3.

Zhu W. "Differential TCM treatment of anovulatory dysfunctional uterine bleeding." *Journal of Traditional Chinese Medicine* 1995;15(4):270-272.

Chapter 10. Drug Treatments

Ang WC, et al. "Effect of hormone replacement therapies and selective estrogen receptor modulators in postmenopausal women with uterine leiomyomas, a literature review." *Climacteric* 2001 Dec;4(4):284-92.

Bianchi S, et al. "Effects on bone mineral density of 12-month goserelin treatment in over 40-year-old women with uterine myomas." *Calcif Tissue Int* 1995 Jul;57(1):78-80.

Carlson KJ, et al. "The Maine Women's Health Study: II. Outcomes of nonsurgical management of leiomyomas." *Obstetrics and Gynecology*, 1994 Apr;83(4):556-72.

Carr BR, Marshburn PB, Weatherall PT, Bradshaw KD, Breslau NA, Byrd W, Roark M, Steinkampf MP. "An evaluation of the effect of gonadotropin-releasing hormone analogs and medroxyprogesterone acetate on uterine leiomyomata volume by magnetic resonance imaging: a prospective, randomized, double blind, placebo-controlled, crossover trial." *J Clin Endocrinol Metab* 1993 May;76(5):1217-23.

Chan WY, et al. "Prostaglandins in primary dysmenorrhea. Comparison of prophylactic and nonprophylactic treatment with ibuprofen and use of oral contraceptives." *Amer J Med* 1981 March;70(3):535-41.

Chavez NF, Stewart EA. "Medical treatment of uterine fibroids." *Clinical Obstetrics and Gynecology* 2001 June;44(2):372-84.

Coutinho EM. "Treatment of large fibroids with high doses of gestrinone." *Gynecol Obstet Invest* l990;30(1):44-7.

Friedman A, et al. Retraction: "Does low-dose combination oral contraceptive use affect uterine size or menstrual flow in premenopausal women with leiomyomas." *Obstetrics and Gynecology* 1995;86(5):728.

Friedman A, et al. Retraction: "Gonatropin-releasing hormone agonist plus estrogen-progestin 'add-back' therapy for endometriosis-related pelvic pain." *Fertility & Sterility* 1996;65(1):211.

Gregoriou O, Konidaris S, Botsis D, Papadias C, Makrakis E, Creatsas G. "Long term effects of Tibolone on postmenopausal women with uterine myomas." *Maturitas* 2001 Oct 31;40(1):95-9.

Hurskainen, R, et al. "Analysis of life and cost-effectiveness of levonorgestrel-releasing intrauterine system versus hysterectomy for treatment of menorrhagia: a randomized trial," *Lancet* 2001 Jan 27;357(9252):273-7.

Iyer V, Farquhar C, Jepson R. "Oral contraceptive pills for heavy menstrual bleeding." *Cochrane Database Syst Rev* 2000; (2): CD000154.

Lethaby AE, Cooke I, Rees M. "Progesterone/progestagen releasing intrauterine systems versus either placebo or any other medication for heavy menstrual bleeding." *Cochrane Database Syst Rev* 2000; (2): CD002126.

Lumbiganon P, et al. "Protective effect of depot-medroxyprogesterone acetate on surgically treated uterine leiomyomas: a multicentre case-control study." *British Journal of Obstetrics and Gynaecology* 1996 Sept;103(9):909-14.

Makarainen L, Ylikorkala O. "Primary and myoma-associated menorrhagia: role of prostaglandins and effects of ibuprofen." *British Journal of Obstetrics and Gynaecology* 1986 Sept;93(9):974-8.

Murphy AA, et al. "Regression of uterine leiomyomata to the antiprogesterone RU486: dose-response effect." *Fertility and Sterility* 1995 Jul;64(1):187-90.

Whelton A. "Renal and related cardiovascular effects of conventional and COX-2-specific NSAIDs and non-NSAID analgesics." *Am J Ther* 2000 Mar;7(2):63-74.

Chapter 11. Uterine Fibroid Embolization

Banovac F, Ascher SM, Jones DA, Black MD, Smith JC, Spies JB. "Magnetic resonance imaging outcome after uterine artery embolization for leiomyomata with use of tris-acryl gelatin microspheres." *J Vasc Interv Radiol* 2002 Jul;13(7):681-8.

Broder MS, Landow WJ, Goodwin SC, Brook RH, Sherbourne CD, Harris K. "An agenda for research into uterine artery embolization: results of an expert panel conference." *JVIR* 2000 Apr;11(4):509-515.

Chrisman HB, Saker MB, Ryu RK, Nemcek AA Jr, Gerbie MV, Milad MP, Smith SJ, Sewall LE, Omary RA, Vogelzang RL. "The impact of uterine fibroid embolization on resumption of menses and ovarian function." *J Vasc Interv Radiol* 2000 Jun;11(6):699-703.

Chrisman HB, Smith SJ, Sterling KM, Vogelzang R, Bonn J, Andrews RT, Worthington-Kirsch RL, Goodwin SC, Lipman JC, Siskin GP, Hovsepian DM. "Uterine fibroid embolization: Developing a clinical service." *Tech Vasc Interv Radiol* 2002 Mar;5(1):67-76.

Coddington CE. "Medical therapy for treatment of uterine fibroids," *Uterine Fibroid Embolization: New Advances in Women's Health Care.* A national conference, Oct. 22-23, 1999, McLean, Virginia.

Goodwin SC, Bonilla SM, Sacks D, Reed RA. Spies JB, Landow WJ, Worthington-Kirsch RL; The Members of the Reporting Standards for Uterine Artery Embolization (UAE) Subcommittee, the Members of the UAE Task Force Standards Subcommittee, and the Members of the SCVIR Technology Assessment Committee. "Reporting standards for uterine artery embolization for the treatment of uterine leiomyomata." *J Vasc Interv Radiol* 2001 Sep;12(9):1011-20.

Goodwin SC, Landow WJ, Matalon TA, Mauro MA, Pomerantz P, Worthington-Kirsch RL. "Opportunity and responsibility: SCVIR's role with uterine artery embolization. Society of Cardiovascular & Interventional Radiology." *J Vasc Interv Radiol* 2000 Apr;11;(4):409-10.

Goodwin SC, McLucas B, Lee M, Chen G, Perrella R, Vedantham S, Muir S, Lai A, Sayre JW, DeLeon M. "Uterine artery embolization for the treatment of uterine leiomyomata midterm results." *J Vasc Interv Radiol* 1999 Oct;10(9):1159-65.

Goodwin SC, Vedantham S, McLucas B, Forno AE, Perrella R. "Preliminary experience with uterine artery embolization for uterine fibroids." *J Vasc Interv Radiol* 1997 Jul-Aug;8(4):517-26.

Goodwin SC, Walker WJ. "Uterine artery embolization for the treatment of uterine fibroids." *Curr Opin Obstet Gynecol* 1998 Aug;10(4):315-20.

Goodwin SC, Wong GCH. "Uterine artery embolization for uterine fibroids: a radiologist's perspective." *Clinical Obstetrics and Gynecology* 2001 Jun;44(2):412-24.

Hutchins FL Jr., Worthington-Kirsch R, Berkowitz RP. "Selective uterine artery embolization as primary treatment for symptomatic leiomyomata uteri." *J Am Assoc Gynecol Laparosc* 1999 Aug;6(3):279-84.

Lai AC, Goodwin SC, Bonilla SM, Lai AP, Yegul T, Vott S, DeLeon M. "Sexual dysfunction after uterine artery embolization." *J Vasc Interv Radiol* 2000 Jun;11(6):755-8.

Lipman JC, Smith SJ, Spies JB, Siskin GP, Machan LS, Bonn J, Worthington-Kirsch RL, Goodwin SC, Hovsepian DM. "Uterine fibroid embolization: Follow-up." *Tech Vasc Interv Radiol* 2002 Mar;5(1):44-55.

McLucas B, Goodwin S, Adler L, Rappaport A, Reed R, Perrella R. "Pregnancy following uterine fibroid embolization." *Int J Gynaecol Obstet* 2001 Jul;74(1):1-7.

McLucas B, Goodwin SC, Adler L, Reed R. "Fatal septicaemia after fibroid embolisation." *Lancet* 1999 Nov 13;354(9191):1730.

McLucas B, Perrella R, Goodwin S, Adler L, Dalrymple J. "Role of uterine artery Doppler flow in fibroid embolization." *J Ultrasound Med* 2002 Feb;21(2):113-20; quiz 122-3.

McLucas B, Reed RA, Goodwin S, Rappaport A, Adler L, Perrella R, Dalrymple J. "Outcomes following unilateral uterine artery embolisation." *Br J Radiol* 2002 Feb;75(890):122-6.

Nikolic B, Spies JB, Abbara S, Goodwin SC. "Ovarian artery supply of uterine fibroids as a cause of treatment failure after uterine artery embolization: a case report." *J Vasc Interv Radiol* 1999 Oct;10(9):1167-70.

Nikolic B, Spies JB, Lundsten MJ, Abbara S. "Patient radiation dose associated with uterine artery embolization." *Radiology* 2000 Jan;214(1): 121-5.

Pelage JP, Le Dref O, Soyer P, Kardache M, Dahan H, Abitbol M, Merland JJ, Ravina JH, Rymer R. "Fibroid-related menorrhagia: treatment with superselective embolization of the uterine arteries and midterm follow-up." *Radiology.* 2000 May;215(2):428-31.

Pelage JP, Walker WJ, Le Dref O. "Re: utility of nonselective abdominal aortography in demonstrating ovarian artery collaterals in patients undergoing uterine artery embolization for fibroids." *J Vasc Interv Radiol* 2002 Jun;13(6):656.

Pron G, Bennett J, Asch M, Sniderman K, Garvin G, Bell S. "The Ontario Multicenter Uterine Fibroid Embolization (UFE) Trial: Part 2—Technical results and effects of experience on uterine artery embolization for fibroids." *Fertility & Sterility.* Submitted.

Pron G, Bennet J, Common A, Wall J, Soucie J, Vilos G. "The Ontario Multicenter Uterine Fibroid Embolization (UFE) Trial: Part 4—Uterine fibroid reduction and symptom relief following uterine artery embolization for fibroids." *Fertility &Sterility.* Submitted.

Pron G, Cohen M, Soucie J, Common A, Simons M, Kachura J. "The Ontario Multicenter Uterine Fibroid Embolization (UFE) Trial: Part 1—Baseline patient characteristics fibroid burden and impact on life.' *Fertility & Sterility.* Submitted.

Pron G, Mocarski E, Vanderburgh L, Kozak R, Zaidi M, Tran C. "The Ontario Multicenter Uterine Fibroid Embolization (UFE) Trial: Part 3—Patient tolerance, hospital stay and recovery following uterine artery embolization for fibroids." *Fertility & Sterility.* Submitted.

Ravina JH, Aymard A, Ciraru-Vigneron N, Ledreff O, Merland JJ. [Arterial embolization of uterine myoma: results apropos of 286 cases]. *J Gynecol Obstet Biol Reprod* (Paris) 2000 May;29(3):272-5.

Ravina JH, Bouret JM, Ciraru-Vigneron N, Repiquet D, Herbreteau D, Aymard A, le Dreff O, Merland JJ, Ferrand J. [Recourse to particular arterial embolization in the treatment of some uterine leiomyoma]. *Bull Acad Natl Med* 1997 Feb;181(2):233-43; discussion 244-6.

Ravina JH, Herbreteau D, Ciraru-Vigneron N, Bouret JM, Houdart E, Aymard A, Merland JJ. "Arterial embolisation to treat uterine myomata." *Lancet* 1995 Sep 9;346(8976):671-2.

Reidy JF, Bradley EA. "Uterine artery embolization for fibroid disease." *Cardio Vascular and Interventional Radiology* 1998 Sept-Oct;21(5):357-60.

Roth AR, Spies JB, Walsh SM, Wood BJ, Gomez-Jorge J, Levy EB. "Pain after uterine artery embolization for leiomyomata: can its severity be predicted and does severity predict outcome?" *J Vasc Interv Radiol* 2000 Sep;11(8):1047-52.

Ryu RK, Chrisman HB, Omary RA, Miljkovic S, Nemcek AA Jr, Saker MB, Resnick S, Carr J, Vogelzang RL. "The vascular impact of uterine artery embolization: prospective sonographic assessment of ovarian arterial circulation." *J Vasc Interv Radiol* 2001 Sep;12(9):1071-4.

Spies JB, Ascher SA, Roth AR, Kim J, Levy EB, Gomez-Jorge J. "Uterine artery embolization for leiomyomata." *Obstet Gynecol* 2001 Jul;98(1):29-34.

Spies J, Niedzwiecki G, Goodwin S, Patel N, Andrews R, Worthington-Kirsch R, Lipman J, Machan L, Sacks D, Sterling K, Lewis C; Task force on Uterine Artery Embolization. Standards Division of Society of Cardiovascular & Interventional Radiology. "Training standards for physicians performing uterine artery embolization for leiomyomata: consensus statement developed by the Task Force on Uterine Artery Embolization and the standards division of the Society of Cardiovascular & Interventional Radiology—August 2000." *J Vasc Interv Radiol* 2001 Jan;12(1):19-21.

Spies JB, Roth AR, Gonsalves SM, Murphy-Skrzyniarz KM. "Ovarian function after uterine artery embolization for leiomyomata: assessment with use of serum follicle stimulating hormone assay." *J Vasc Interv Radiol* 2001 Apr;12(4):437-42.

Spies JB, Roth AR, Jha RC, Gomez-Jorge J, Levy EB, Chang TC, Ascher SA. "Leiomyomata treated with uterine artery embolization: factors associated with successful symptom and imaging outcome." *Radiology* 2002 Jan;222(1):45-52.

Spies JB, Scialli AR, Jha RC, Imaoka I, Ascher SM, Fraga VM, Barth KH. "Initial results from uterine fibroid embolization for symptomatic leiomyomata." *J Vase Interv Radiol* 1999 Oct;10(9):1149-57.

Sterling KM, Vogelzang RL, Chrisman HB, Worthington-Kirsch RL, Machan LS, Goodwin SC, Andrews RT, Hovsepian DM, Smith SJ, Bonn J. "Uterine fibroid embolization: Management of complications." *Tech Vasc Interv Radiol* 2002 Mar;5(1):56-66.

Subramanian S, Spies JB. "Uterine artery embolization for leiomyomata: resource use and cost estimation." *J Vasc Interv Radiol* 2001 May;12(5):571-4.

Vedantham S, Goodwin SC, McLucas B, Lee M, Perrella R, Forno AE, DeLeon M. "Uterine artery embolization for fibroids: considerations in patient selection and clinical follow-up." *Medscape Womens Health* 1999 Oct;4(5):2.

Vedantham S, Sterling KM, Goodwin SC, Spies JB, Shlansky-Goldberg R, Worthington-Kirsch RL, Andrews RT, Hovsepian DM, Smith SJ, Chrisman HB. "Uterine fibroid embolization: Preprocedure assessment." *Tech Vasc Interv Radiol* 2002 Mar;5(1):2-16.

Vott S, Bonilla SM, Goodwin SC, Chen G, Wong GC, Lai A. Yegul T, DeLeon M. "CT findings after uterine artery embolization." *J Comput Assist Tomogr* 2000 Nov-Dec;24(6):846-8.

Watson GM, Walker WJ. "Uterine artery embolisation for the treatment of symptomatic fibroids in 114 women: reduction in size of the fibroids and women's views of the success of the treatment." *BJOG* 2002 Feb;109(2):129-35.

Wong GC, et al. "Uterine artery embolization: a minimally invasive technique for the treatment of uterine fibroids." *Journal of Women's Health & Gender-Based Medicine* 2000;9(6):357-362.

Wong GC, Muir SJ, Lai AP, Goodwin SC. "Uterine artery embolization: a minimally invasive technique for the treatment of uterine fibroids." *J Womens Health Gend Based Med* 2000 May;9(4):357-62.

Worthington-Kirsch RL, et al. "Uterine arterial embolization for the management of leiomyomas: quality-of-life assessment and clinical response." *Vascular and Interventional Radiology* 1998 Sept;208:625-9.

Worthington-Kirsch RL, Andrews RT, Siskin GP, Shlansky-Goldberg R, Lipman JC, Goodwin SC, Bonn J, Hovsepian DM. "Uterine fibroid embolization: Technical aspects." *Tech Vasc Interv Radiol* 2002 Mar;5(1):17-34.

Worthington-Kirsch R, Fueredi G, Goodwin S, Machan L, Niedzwiecki G, Reidy J, Spies J, Walker W. "Polyvinyl alcohol particle size for uterine artery embolization." *Radiology* 2001 Feb;218(2):605-6.

Chapter 12. Myomectomy

Berkeley AS, DeCherney AH, Polan ML. "Abdominal myomectomy and subsequent fertility." *Surg Gynecol Obstet* 1983 Mar;156(3):319-22.

Doridot V, Dubuisson JB, Chapron C, Fauconnier A, Babaki-Fard K. "Recurrence of leiomyomata after laparoscopic myomectomy." *J Am Assoc Gynecol Laparosc* 2001 Nov;8(4):495-500.

Farquhar C, Vandekerckhove P, Watson A, Vail A, Wiseman D. "Barrier agents for preventing adhesions after surgery for subfertility." *Cochrane Database Syst Rev* 2000; (2): CD000475.

Fauconnier A, Chapron C, Babaki-Fard K, Dubuisson JB. "Recurrence of leiomyomata after myomectomy." *Hum Reprod Update* 2000 Nov-Dec;6(6):595-602.

Guarnaccia MS, Rein MS. "Traditional surgical approaches to uterine fibroids: abdominal myomectomy and hysterectomy." *Clinical Obstetrics and Gynecology* 2001 June;44(2):385-400.

Hutchins FL Jr. "A randomized comparison of vasopressin and tourniquet as hemostatic agents during myomectomy." *Obstet Gynecol* 1996 Oct;88(4 Pt 1):639-40.

Lethaby A, Shepperd S, Cooke I, Farquhar C. "Endometrial resection and ablation versus hysterectomy for heavy menstrual bleeding." *Cochrane Database Syst Rev* 2000; (2):CD000329.

Magdy PM, Rajendras SS. "Laparoscopic approaches to uterine leiomyomas." *Clinical Obstetrics and Gynecology* June 2001.

"Management of Uterine Fibroids." Evidence Report No. 34, AHRQ publication No. 01-E051. January 2001. Agency for Healthcare Research and Quality, Rockville, MD.

Subramanian S, Clark MA, Isaacson K. "Outcome and resource use associated with myomectomy." *Obstet Gynecol* 2001 Oct;98(4):583-7.

Verkauf BS. "Myomectomy for fertility enhancement and preservation." *Fertil Steril* 1992 Jul;58(1):1-15.

Chapter 13. Hysterectomy

Akkad AA, et al. "Abnormal uterine bleeding on hormone replacement: the importance of intrauterine structural abnormalities." *Obstetrics and Gynecology* 1995 Sept;86(3):330-4.

Bernstein SJ, McGlynn EA, Siu AL, Roth CP, Sherwood MJ, Keesey JW, Kosecoff J, Hicks NR, Brook RH. "The appropriateness of hysterectomy. A comparison of care in seven health plans." Health Maintenance Organization Quality of Care Consortium. *JAMA* 1993 May 12;269 (18):2398-402.

Broder MS, et al. "The appropriateness of recommendations for hysterectomy." *Obstet Gynecol* 2000 Feb; 95(2):199-205.

Carlson KJ, et al. "The Maine Women's Health Study: I. Outcomes of hysterectomy." *Obstetrics and Gynecology* 1994 Apr; 83(4)556-65.

D'esopo A. "Hysterectomy when the uterus is grossly normal." *Am J Obstet Gynecol* 1962 Jan:113-122.

Hulley S, et al. "Randomized trial of estrogen plus progestin for secondary prevention of coronary heart disease in postmenopausal women." *Journal of the American Medical Association* 1998 Aug 19;280(7):605-13.

Kilkku P, et al. "Supravaginal uterine amputation vs. Hysterectomy." *Acta Obstet Gynecol Scan* 1983;62(2):141-52.

"Management of Uterine Fibroids." Evidence Report No. 34, AHRQ publication No. 01-E051. January 2001. Agency for Healthcare Research and Quality, Rockville, MD.

Sener AB, et al. "The effects of hormone replacement therapy on uterine fibroids in postmenopausal women." *Fertility & Sterility* 1996 Feb;65(2):354-7.

Sloan D. "The emotional and psychosexual aspects of hysterectomy."

American Journal of Obstetrics and Gynecology 1978 July 15;131(6):598-605.

Strauss B, et al. "Psychiatric and sexual sequelae of hysterectomy—a comparison of different surgical methods." *Geburtshilfe Frauenheilkd* 1996 Sept;56(9):473-81.

Thakar R, et al. "Bladder, bowel and sexual function after hysterectomy for benign conditions." *British Journal of Obstetrics and Gynaecology* 1997 Sept;104(9):983-7.

Thakar R, Ayers S, Clarkson P, Stanton S, Manyonda I. "Outcomes after total versus subtotal abdominal hysterectomy." *N Engl J Med.* 2002 Oct 24;347(17):1360-2.

Chapter 14. Into the Future

Burroughs KD, et al. "Regulation of apoptosis in uterine leiomyomata." *Endocrinology* 1997 July;138(7):3056-64.

Christman GM, McCarthy JD. "Gene therapy and uterine leiomyomas." *Clinical Obstetrics and Gynecology* 2001 June;77(4):645-57.

Donnez J, Squifflet J, Polet R, Nisolle M. "Laparoscopic myolysis." *Hum Reprod Update* 2000 Nov-Dec;6(6):609-13.

Goldfarb HA. "Combining myoma coagulation with endometrial ablation/resection reduces subsequent surgery rates." *JSLS* 1999 Oct-Dec;3(4):253-60.

Goldfarb HA. "Myoma coagulation (myolysis)." *Obstet Gynecol Clin North Am* 2000 June;27(2):421-30.

Goldfarb HA. "A review of 35 endometrial ablations using the Nd:YAG laser for recurrent menometrorrhagia." *Obstetrics and Gynecology* 1990 Nov;(5 Pt 5)833-5.

Howe SR, et al. "Rodent model of reproductive tract leiomyomata. Establishments and characterization of tumor-derived cell lines." *American Journal of Pathology* 1995 Jun;146(6):1568-79.

Kettel LM, Murphy AA, Morales AJ, Yen SS. "Clinical efficacy of the antiprogesterone RU486 in the treatment of endometriosis and uterine fibroids." *Hum Reprod* 1994 Jun;9 Suppl 1:116-20.

Lee BS, et al. "Pirfenidone: a novel pharmacological agent that inhibits leiomyoma cell proliferation and collagen production." *Journal of Clinical Endocrinology and Metabolism* 1998 Jan;83(1):219-23.

Nisolle M, Smets M, Malvaux V, Anaf V, Donnez J. "Laparoscopic myoly-sis with the Nd:YAG laser." *J Gynecol Surg* 1993 Summer;9(2):95-9.

Soderstrom R. "Endometrial ablation—where we've been; where we're going." *Contemporary Ob/Gyn* 2000;4:61-67.

Stewart EA, Nowak RA. "New concepts in the treatment of uterine leiomy-omas." *Obstetrics and Gynecolog,* 1998 Oct;92(4 Pt 1):624-7.

"Ultrasound surgery shrinks symptomatic uterine fibroids," *Reuters,* November 26, 2001.

"What is the Gamma Knife Radiosurgery Center?" Wake Forest University. Website: www.wfubmc.edu/surg-sci/ns/gkc.html.

Zreik TG, Rutherford TJ, Palter SF, Troiano RN, Williams E, Brown JM, Olive DL. "Cryomyolysis, a new procedure for the conservative treatment of uterine fibroids." *J Am Assoc Gynecol Laparosc* 1998 Feb;5(1):33-8.

Additional Resources

BOOKS

Beckmann, C., et al., *Obstetrics and Gynecology.* Baltimore: Williams & Wilkins, 1998.

Dionne, Carla, *Sex, Lies and the Truth about Uterine Fibroids: A Journey from Diagnosis to Treatment to Renewed Good Health.* New York: Avery, Penguin Putnam: 2001.

Hudson, Tori, M.D., *Women's Encyclopedia of Natural Medicine: Alternative Therapies and Integrative Medicine.* Los Angeles: Keats Publishing.

Lark, Susan, M.D., *Fibroid Tumors & Endometriosis Self-Help Book.* Berkeley, CA: Celestial Arts, 1995.

Lark, Susan, M.D., and James A. Richards, M.B.A., *The Chemistry of Success: Six Secrets of Peak Performance.* San Francisco: Bay Books, 2000.

Lee, John R, M.D., with Virginia Hopkins. *What Your Doctor May Not Tell You about Menopause: The Breakthrough Book on Natural Progesterone.* New York: Warner Books, 1996.

Love, Susan, M.D., and Karen Lindsey, *Dr. Susan Love's Hormone Book: Making Informed Choices about Menopause.* New York: Random House, 1997.

Moore, J.G., Hacker, N.F., and Schmitt, W. *Essentials of Obstetrics and Gynecology.* Philadelphia: W.B. Saunders, 1998.

Morgan, Susanne, Ph.D., *Coping with a Hysterectomy: Your Own Chice, Your Own Solutions*, Rev. Edition, New York: Plume, 1985.

Murray, Michael and Joseph Pizzorno, *Encyclopedia of Natural Medicine*, Rev. 2nd Edition, Rocklin, CA: Prima Publishing, 1998.

Parker, William H., M.D., with Rachel L. Parker, and contributions by Ingrid A. Rodi, M.D., and Amy E. Rosenman, M.D., *A Gynecologist's Second Opinion: The Questions and Answers You Need to Take Charge of Your Health.* New York: Plume/Penguin, 1996.

Shealy, Norman C., ed., *The Illustrated Encyclopedia of Natural Remedies.* Boston: Element Books, 1998.

Siegal, D.L., et al., *The New Ourselves, Growing Older: Women Aging with Knowledge and Power.* Boston Women's Health Collective. New York: Touchstone/Simon & Schuster, 1994.

Strausz, Ivan K., M.D., *You Don't Need a Hysterectomy: New and Effective Ways of Avoiding Major Surgery,* 2nd ed. Cambridge, MA: Perseus Publishing, 2001.

Stringer, Nelson H., M.D., *Uterine Fibroids: What Every Woman Needs to Know.* Glenville, IL: Physicians and Scientists Publishing, 1996.

Thompson, J.A., Te Linde, R.W., and Rock, J.D., *Te Linde's Operative Gynecology.* Philadelphia: Lippincott-Raven, 1997.

West, Stanley with Paula Dranov, *The Hysterectomy Hoax.* New York: Doubleday, 1995.

Westcott, Patsy and Leyardia Black, N.D., *Alternative Health Care for Women: A Woman's Guide to Self-Help Treatments and Natural Therapies.* Rochester, VT: Healing Arts Press, 1987.

ORGANIZATIONS

American Association of Gynecologic Laparoscopists
13021 Florence Avenue

Santa Fe Springs, CA 90670
Phone: (800) 554-AAGL
Internet: www.aagl.com

American Association of Naturopathic Physicians
3201 New Mexico Avenue NW, Suite 350
Washington, D.C. 20016
Phone: (866) 538-2267
Internet: www.naturopathic.org

American Association of Sex Educators, Counselors, and Therapists
P.O. Box 5488
Richmond, VA 23220-0488
Internet: www.aasect.org

American Cancer Society
1559 Clifton Road, NE
Atlanta, GA 30329
Phone: (800) ACS-2345
Internet: www.cancer.org

American College of Obstetricians and Gynecologists
409 12th Street, SW; P.O. Box 96920
Washington, DC 20090-6920
Phone: (202) 863-2518
Internet: www.acog.org

American Society of Anesthesiologists
520 N. Northwest Highway
Park Ridge, IL 60068-2573
Phone: (847) 825-5586
Internet: www.asahq.org

American Society for Reproductive Medicine
1209 Montgomery Highway
Birmingham, AL 35216-2809
Phone: (205) 978-5000
Internet: www.asrm.org

American Urogynecologic Association
2025 M Street, NW, Suite 800

Washington, DC 20036
Phone: (202) 367-1167
E-mail: augs@dc.sba.com
Internet www.augs.org

Center for Uterine Fibroids
Brigham and Women's Hospital
Departments of Obstetrics/Gynecology
623 Thorn Building
20 Shattuck Street
Boston, Massachusetts 02115
Phone: (800) 722-5520, Ext. 80081
Internet: www.fibroids.net

Endometriosis Association
8585 North 76th Place
Milwaukee, WI 53223
Phone: (414) 355-2200; (800) 992-3636 in North America and
Caribbean
Internet: www.endometriosisassn.org/

National Black Women's Health Project
600 Pennsylvania Avenue, SE #310
Washington, DC 20003
Phone: (202)543-9311
Internet: www.nbwhp.org

National Cancer Institute
NCI Public Inquiries Office, Suite 3036A
6116 Executive Boulevard, MSC 8322
Bethesda, MD 20892-8322
Phone: (800) 4-CANCER
Internet: www.nci.nih.gov

National Center for Alternative and Complementary Medicine
P.O. Box 8218
Silver Spring, MD 20907
Phone: (888) 644-6226
Internet: www.ncam.nih.gov

National Certification Commission for Acupuncture and Oriental Medicine
11 Canal Center Plaza, Suite 300
Alexandria, VA 22314
Phone: (705) 548-9004
Internet: www.nccaom.org

National Osteoporosis Foundation
1232 22nd Street NW
Washington, DC 20037
Phone: (800) 223-9994
Internet: www.nof.org

National Uterine Fibroids Foundation
P.O. Box 9688
Colorado Springs, CO 80932-0688
Phone: (877) 553-NUFF (6833); (719) 633-3454
E-mail: info@NUFF.org
Internet: www.NUFF.org

National Women's Health Information Center (NWHIC)
8550 Arlington Boulevard, Suite 300
Fairfax, VA 22031
Phone: (800) 994-9662
Internet: www.4woman.gov

National Women's Health Network
514 10th Street, NW, Suite 400
Washington, DC 20004
Phone: (202) 628-7814 (health info); (202) 347-1140
Internet: www.womenshealthnetwork.org

North American Menopause Society
P.O. Box 94527
Cleveland, OH 44101
Phone: (440) 442-7550
Internet: www.menopause.org

Sexuality Information and Education Council of the United States
130 W. 42nd Street, Suite 350

New York, NY 10036
Phone: (212) 819-9770
Internet: www.siecus.org

Society of Interventional Radiology
10201 Lee Highway, #500
Fairfax, VA 22030
Phone: (800) 488-7284; (703) 691-1805
Internet: www.sirweb.org

Women's Cancer Resource Center
5741 Telegraph Avenue
Oakland, CA 94609
Phone: (510) 548-9286
Internet: www.wcrc.org

WEBSITES

groups.yahoo.com/group/uterinefibroids
Uterine fibroids research and support e-mail-based group sponsored by
the National Uterine Fibroids Foundation.

groups.yahoo.com/group/embo
Uterine fibroid embolization e-mail-based support group.

www.ama-assn.org/special/womh
Journal of the American Medical Association information site designed as a
resource for doctors and other health professionals.

www.abms.org
American Board of Medical Specialties can check board certifications of
any medical doctor.

www.healthfinder.gov/
Easy search of health information on this site sponsored by the U.S.
Department of Health and Human Services.

www.ncbi.nlm.nih.gov/PubMed/
Government site provides free access to Medline, a scientific database that
may be searched for medical journal abstracts and article citations.

www.findings.net/sans-uteri.html
Online support group for women considering a hysterectomy or recovering from one.

www.uterinefibroids.com
Uterine Fibroids website of Carla Dionne, author of *Sex, Lies and Uterine Fibroids*.

www.gynsecondopinion.com
William Parker, M.D. (CA)

www.fda.gov
Food and Drug Administration home page; can be searched for information about particular drugs.

groups.yahoo.com/group/adenomyosis
Adenomyosis e-mail-based support group.

www.fibroids.net
Brigham and Women's Hospital's Ob/Gyn Department (MA)

www.fibroidtreatment.com
Scott Goodwin, M.D. (CA)

www.fibroidoptions.com
Georgetown University Medical Center Department of Radiology and James Spies, M.D. (Washington, DC)

www.fibroidregistry.org
Society of Interventional Radiology

www.sirweb.org
Society of Interventional Radiology

Index

About the Authors

Scott G. Goodwin, M.D., is best known for introducing uterine artery embolization for the treatment of uterine fibroids in the United States. He has been asked to lecture on this topic nationally and internationally over one hundred times. Dr. Goodwin graduated magna cum laude from UCLA with departmental honors and finished in the top 15 percent of his class at Harvard Medical School. His residency and fellowship were completed at UCLA, and he is double boarded in diagnostic radiology and vascular and interventional radiology. Multiple medical societies count him as a member, and he was recently elected Fellow of the Society of Interventional Radiology. Notable service includes chief of vascular and interventional radiology at UCLA for seven years and chairman and professor of radiology at Wayne State University in the 2001–2002 academic year. He is currently chief of imaging at the Greater Los Angeles Veterans Administration Health Care System in West Los Angeles and is professor of radiology at UCLA. He continues to provide uterine fibroid embolization at Terran Medical Corporation in Los Angeles, California, where he is chief of interventional radiology.

Michael S. Broder, M.D., M.S.H.S., is an assistant professor of obstetrics and gynecology at the UCLA School of Medicine. He has extensive research training and has served as a consultant to the RAND Corporation (a research think tank in Santa Monica, California) since 1996. He has earned a listing in Who's Who in America, 2001.

Dr. Broder's work has been published in the *Los Angeles*

Times, as well as in scientific publications, including the *Journal of the American Medical Association*, *Obstetrics & Gynecology*, *Health Services Research*, the *Western Journal of Medicine*, and the *Journal of Vascular and Interventional Radiology*. His research has been cited in numerous newspapers and magazines, including *Health*, *Prevention*, *Parenting*, and *Family Circle*. He is a frequent public speaker on women's health issues. Dr. Broder has also studied the overuse of hysterectomy to treat gynecologic problems. He is on the board of the National Uterine Fibroids Foundation, a group dedicated to helping women with uterine fibroids.

A